AF604155

Beyond Neglect: Leveraging Technology for Effective NTD Control in Africa

Navya

Copyright © 2024 by Navya

All rights reserved. No part of this book may be reproduced in any manner whatso-ever without written permission except in the case of brief quotations embodied in critical articles and reviews.

First Printing, 2024

Table of Contents

1 Introduction

Increasingly health departments around the world, and also in Africa, are recognizing the importance and potential impact of electronic health information systems to support decision making on various levels. It is assumed that the use of ICT would lead to greater efficiency in the use of resources and have the potential to transform healthcare systems for better service delivery. Most health departments have already installed integrated electronic reporting systems for the major diseases and health indicators. Even in Africa, many countries including Kenya, Ghana and Sierra Leone have, for instance, adopted the District Health Information System (DHIS2) platform. Some are even experimenting with m-Health tools for data collection, for instance, the various m-Health initiatives in Kenya and Ethiopia linked to community volunteers in the HIV care sector, maternal and child health, and e-learning.

However, some sectors, for instance, the Neglected Tropical Diseases Sector and in particular Leprosy, have traditionally been neglected for a variety of reasons and are still dependent on fragmented paper-based systems for data collection around the world.

Recently the World Health Organization (WHO) and others have initiated the development of m-Health tools based on the DHIS2 platform to modernize the Case Managed Neglected Tropical Diseases (CM-NTD) notification system and also allow for the mapping of these diseases. The purpose of this study was to identify factors that would enhance or impede the integration of these electronic health information systems for the Case Managed Neglected Tropical Diseases (CM-NTDs) sector in Mozambique and make a positive contribution to Knowledge Management (KM) in this somewhat unique sector.

This deductive study used cycles in a Soft Systems Methodology (Action Research) approach during the implementation of such a system within the Mozambique context, recognizing the many unstructured community and institutional relationships that have an impact on the outcomes of this complex disease.

Problem statement and Research Question

Leprosy has been around for thousands of years. It is a slow and patient disease with an incubation period of 5 years or longer usually targeting the poorest of the poor, mainly in countries where people can least afford the burden of disability and the stigma that it causes. Societies have dealt with it in various ways over the millennia in attempts to prevent the disease and its spread in communities. Mostly, it has involved isolating people from their communities and shutting them away on islands or secluded areas. Only in relatively recent times from the 1970´s and 80´s onward has a real cure been available. This has led to new treatment strategies and enabled the people with leprosy to return to their communities.

As part of this strategy, leprosy was made a notifiable disease in an effort to track its spread as well as the effects of the efforts to eradicate the disease. This took the form of book-based Leprosy registers that were filled-in by the diagnosing healthcare worker; whereafter, information was aggregated by health departments and the WHO on various levels. Armed with this instrument and the WHO backed and sponsored treatment regimes, there was an expectation that leprosy could finally be beaten.

After forty years of intense leprosy control activities across the world and notwithstanding the achievement of attaining a prevalence of less than 1 case per 10,000 of the population in most leprosy endemic countries, it became apparent however that effective antibiotic treatment alone was not sufficient to stop leprosy. Over the past 10 years as more evidence from various endemic regions across the world became available, it indicated that the transmission of Leprosy was still continuing (Smith, Aerts, Kita, & Virmond, 2016) .

The Leprosy community realized that it had to adapt once again in its approach to address this problem, before the gains that have been made over the past 40 years were wiped out by the slow creeping progress of the disease. Health Departments across the world, however, having achieved a low prevalence of leprosy did not consider it a public health problem any longer. Leprosy was grouped as one of the many Case Managed Neglected Tropical Diseases (CM-NTDs) that poorer health departments have to deal with, and as it is a relatively small disease, resources were diverted elsewhere, and delivery and control systems stagnated (Smith, van Brakel, Gillis, Saunderson, & Richardus, 2015).

One of the results of the failing control systems of leprosy was that the information systems became unreliable. In Mozambique for example at the time of writing this study the information was based on book leprosy registers and various versions of aggregated Excel tables. As staff and resources for Leprosy were diverted to other programs, the shortcomings of the book-based information system was also compounded as the accuracy of the data could no longer be verified.

Fortunately, over the past 40 years there have been many other developments in the delivery and control systems of the healthcare sector. In particular, over the past 15 years, there have been major developments in the availability of information technology able to benefit health outcomes for patients and contributing to a greater epidemiological understanding of diseases (Deloitte, 2015). The advantages and disadvantages of electronic health information systems have also become apparent in many other parts of the health sector where there have been great expectations for the positive impact of modern communication (Collins-Higgins et al., 2015), but also many failures of large and expensive systems (Heeks, 1998).

For the fight against leprosy, the time has come to learn some lessons from the failed attempts of the past and to find better ways to design and implement an information system for Leprosy in this specific context. As the disease of Leprosy is currently caught in the doldrums of strategic uncertainty, the need for accurate and more detailed epidemiological information is more pressing in order to give more momentum and focus to the innovative ways in which the healthcare sector and communities affected by leprosy are mobilized to stop the disease. It is not just about gathering data, but increasingly about how a wider group of actors can interact with the information and use the knowledge in productive ways in order to drive back this ancient disease.

In this context the following research question was developed:

What factors would contribute to the successful implementation of a health information system for CM-NTDs in order to improve Knowledge Management within the wider NTD care system?

We have a strong indication from the literature of the importance of knowledge management for the improvement of health services (Amori, Chindlund, & Zipperer, 2016). There are also many examples where the integration of Knowledge Management systems were not successful (Littlejohns, 2003). It is therefore important that we learn about the integration of these systems into a context where they are not native, like Africa, and where there can be a bigger risk of them failing. The term Knowledge Management is used within a variety of disciplines and fields, including business, the healthcare sector and information systems. In general it is seen as a process where knowledge and information is created, shared and used (Girard & Girard, 2015). In this study we will attempt to move our focus away from just the implementation of a health information system towards the ultimate goal of capturing and sharing that knowledge and information so that it can influence program implementation and ultimately patient outcomes.

At the time of writing, the WHO was developing a DHIS2-based health information platform and the adaptation and contextualization of this instrument in the Mozambique context is the basis of this study.

The District Health Information Software 2 (DHIS2) is an open source, web-based health management information system (HMIS) platform. It is the world's largest HMIS platform which is being used in many low and middle income countries (Braa & Sahay, 2017).

These tools and the lessons learned could be applied in various other countries to support the NTD programs. An added objective of the proposed study would be to develop an approach to contextualizing this particular tool for the CM-NTD service sector and identify specific issues that could contribute to improved knowledge management in the long-run. Both the information system prototype, as well as our approach to integrating it could be adapted and improved through various iterations of an Action Research process in various contexts over time and can be useful for developing a model for information system development in these contexts.

As in most societies, the growth of mobile networks as well as social networking is bringing changes to the way healthcare workers do their jobs (Long, Pariyo, & Kallander, 2018) and it opens many new possibilities for social mobilization and community involvement in service provision. Through the implementation of the study we will get an insight into how Mozambique society is changing and how the engagement of healthcare workers with mobile technology can contribute to better service delivery.

2 Literature Review

The literature review is structured in the following way:

2.1 The Neglected Tropical Diseases care system.

2.2 The specific challenges of Leprosy within the Neglected Tropical Diseases care system.

2.3 The use of Health information systems to support the Neglected Tropical diseases care sector.

2.4 Perspectives on Knowledge Management and its importance in the healthcare and NTD contexts.

2.5 The importance of Information and Communication technology for knowledge management.

2.6 The importance of the bigger knowledge management goals when introducing Information and communication technologies in the healthcare and NTD contexts.

2.7 Theories on the adoption of innovations relevant to health information system implementation.

2.8 Health information systems implementation and Knowledge Management in the African and Mozambique contexts.

2.1 The neglected tropical diseases care system

"Neglected tropical diseases (NTDs) encompass 17 viral, bacterial and parasitic diseases that occur solely, or principally in tropical regions. They are often termed 'neglected' as the people who are most affected are the poorest populations living in rural areas, urban slums and conflict zones. Nearly half of the burden of NTDs is believed to occur in the African Region. These diseases lead to disabilities, cause discrimination within communities, and promote the ongoing cycle of poverty" (WORLD HEALTH ORGANISATION, 2016)

The burden and impact of NTDs especially in Africa is probably severely underestimated because of their adverse effects on pregnancy outcomes, early child development and even agricultural worker productivity in the poorest populations in sub-Sahara Africa (Hotez & Kamath, 2009).

"The WHO recommends a combination of five strategies for the prevention and control of NTDs, which are applied according to the epidemiology of the specific NTD. The strategies are preventive

chemotherapy (PCT); intensified case-management; vector control; safe water, sanitation and hygiene; and veterinary public health" (Samuels & Pose, 2013 p. 2)

Over the past decade, preventative chemotherapy has especially received much attention and investment. With the donation of drugs for Mass Drug Administration (MDA) campaigns, much progress has been made in the fight against diseases like schistosomiasis, intestinal parasites and lymphatic filariasis, as they occur together in the same geographical localities and have a high prevalence, which allows for combined country wide strategies.

Some NTDs are called Case Managed NTDs (CM-NTDs) as they need individual diagnosis and often specialized case by case treatment. CM-NTDs usually have a lower prevalence and pose unique challenges in term of diagnosis, treatment and longer-term rehabilitation as they often cause a high degree of disability, for example, Buruli ulcer and Leprosy. In Mozambique, the most common CM-NTDs are Lymphedema and Hydrocele (both caused by Lymphatic Filariasis), Leprosy, and Trachoma.

These diseases have high demands in terms of needed resources, time, expertise and coordination for the health department to manage them effectively. They require specialized clinical skills to diagnose, long treatment regimens, and specialized interventions to manage complications, for instance surgery. These resources, especially the clinical knowledge and skills are often lacking within the context that NTDs are found. The longer treatment cycles and relatively low prevalence have also made it less attractive for international funders to invest in the CM-NTDs. These characteristics of especially CM-NTDs like the clinical skills needed for diagnosis, the long-term treatment cycles, and need for followup, emphasise the need for good record keeping and the maintenance of knowledge within this care system. Furthermore there are concerns that big mass drug administration campaigns may undermine healthcare systems that are already fragile in countries with limited resources and implementation capacity (Marchal et al., 2011). In NTD care it is also important to address the social aspects of the diseases as well as the wider health systems context in order to properly serve the poorest of the poor (Meheus, Rijal, Lutumba, Hendrickx, & Boelaert, 2012). The interface between the NTD disease management programs and general health services brings with it some unique challenges.

2.2 The specific challenges of Leprosy within the neglected tropical diseases care system

Leprosy, also known as "Hansen's disease", is a chronic disease caused by the bacteria Mycobacterium leprae which primarily affects the skin and peripheral nerves (Lockwood, 2007). It spreads probably through droplet spread as nasal secretions of especially lepromatous cases can contain millions of viable bacteria (Bhat & Prakash, 2012). The incubation time can be notoriously long, from 3 years up to 30 years have been documented. The disease has a wide spectrum of clinical presentation depending mostly on the immunological response of the host to the infection. It is further exacerbated by various possible complications causing further nerve damage which increases the possibility to develop disabilities due to the disease. Treatment has been available since the 1980s and consists of a combination of various antibiotics including Rifampicine, Dapsone and Clofazimine. Depending on the level of disease, the treatment duration is usually between 6 to 12 months of daily antibiotics. Except for the pharmacological treatment, various other interventions may be needed to treat already existing disability or to prevent new disabilities from developing. Leprosy often has a social dimension as well with people suffering from social exclusion due to the effects of stigma or self-stigma. The annual detection rate of leprosy worldwide is currently just over 200'000 new cases per year and has maintained this level for quite a number of years already (Britton, 2017).

In a review of the recent advances in the clinical and laboratory knowledge in the field of leprosy, Scollard et al., (2006) concluded that even though the number of registered cases of leprosy have been declining, the actual case burden have likely stayed the same for the past two decades. This highlights the need for continued emphasis on research and also the clinical and operational disease management in the field. Even if a highly effective vaccine was produced, or if accurate early diagnostic tools were readily available, it would still pose enormous challenges in roll-out strategies as well as screening of apparent asymptomatic contacts and populations. These tools are unfortunately still not available, and the continued task of providing good diagnostic and clinical care still falls with the program implementers. Leprosy control programs across the world have had a battle to make their voices heard within the wider health concerns in poorer countries. Due to increased pressure on health departments to reduce the prevalence of leprosy, many have used alternative ways to manipulate the statistics without really reducing the burden of the disease. These factors have now called into question the quality of the worldwide statistics on leprosy (Burki, 2009).

Leprosy will unfortunately still be around for a long time, but it is crucial that the scope and distribution of the disease be well understood so that political and financial resources can be mobilized to stop the disease. Health information systems related to leprosy needs to be robust enough to withstand international scrutiny and verification so that disease control programs can work with credibility.

2.3 The use of health information systems to support the neglected tropical diseases care sector

Information systems to support the implementation of the Global Neglected tropical diseases program has been very contextual and vertical in nature. This is largely due to the large scale of these diseases as well as to the specific characteristics and information needs of each of the many diseases included as neglected tropical diseases. The global program for the elimination of Lymphatic Filariasis has for instance recommended that all endemic countries should be collecting and reporting data on morbidity management by the end of 2014 (WHO, 2013). National health departments have till now not had the operational capacity to measure much more than aggregate data from the mass drug administration campaigns. Some of the international NGOs working in the NTD field has taken up the challenge and have experimented with a variety of m-health tools for instance SMS and Android based platforms (King et al., 2013) to capture data on for instance lymphoedema and hydrocoele. They have often involved community healthcare workers and other non-government staff to collect and verify data and have demonstrated mostly promising results (Stanton et al., 2015). In a large scale community survey a comparison was for instance made between a paper based survey and the results from an Android application based system. Costs incurred during the process was roughly the same, but time was saved by the electronic survey and the results were immediately available (King et al., 2013). The geographical coordinates collected from the Android based devises was much more accurate than coordinated transcribed on a paper

form.
The vertical nature and disease specific design of these systems as well as a lack of data analysis capacity in low and middle income countries (Nabyonga-Orem, 2017) could however prevent their continued use or prevent health departments from accepting the validity of the results.

Leprosy care has been around for a long time and was included as a vertical program in most health departments in endemic countries long before it was classified as a neglected tropical disease. From early on it was a notifiable disease so some form of register was necessary to track the spread of the disease. The WHO was heavily involved from the start with the involvement of a handful of NGOs specializing in leprosy care. As treatment became available in the 1980's an initiative was launched to develop standardised leprosy notification forms for notification and record keeping of individual patients. This simplified information system for leprosy (OMSLEP) was tested in 15 countries (Lechat, Misson, Walter, Seal, & Sansarricq, 1980) and formed the basis for the leprosy paper based health information system still in use in many leprosy endemic countries. The system consisted of an individual patient record form, patient followup forms for periodic re-evaluations as well as annual statistics forms for the calculation and notification of periodic aggregate data. As data began to be shared between various countries, it became increasingly necessary to standardize the indicators used for tracking the various treatment outcomes and disease trends in leprosy which led to improvements in the quality of care in various control programs (Yellapurkar, n.d.).

Over the subsequent years, various attempts have been made to improve the record keeping and data management systems for leprosy, but not all have been documented. With greater availability of computers the simple Excel spreadsheet has probably been the most used instrument in all endemic countries to capture aggregate data or to share data between levels in the healthcare hierarchy. Shortly after the OMSLEP system were put into practice a similar computerized system was piloted in India using a dBase III database. It was observed that computerized reports were more useful for monitoring both at microlevel as well as macrolevel. Staff doing the data reporting also found that they saved the time previously spent preparing monthly progress reports manually. Overall the staff working with the system had a positive experience and enjoyed learning a new technology

(Revankar, Goyal, & Sorensen, 1989). Even though there were good experiences and positive expectations of these systems they did not stand the test of time and little information could be found as to why the positive outcomes were not followed through and implemented on the longer term.

Other instruments used was EpiInfo and SMS based systems (Castro, 2013) but none of these managed to find a sustainable user base. In an attempt to modernise the leprosy information system in Indonesia, an evaluation was done of the system used in Taiwan, where leprosy was successfully eradicated. Indonesia still ranks third after India and Brasil as the country with the highest leprosy burden worldwide. It was noted that not only the information system alone, but especially the interaction between the information and the case management and followup systems were important to successfully control the disease. The system in Taiwan seemed to be better integrated in the national information system and used the national identity number to register patients and to link them to their treatment followup observer (Rachmani & Hsu, 2013). An electronic health information system was subsequently introduced for leprosy in Indonesia, but due to the size of the population and the logistical difficulties to reach its population, the road has been much more difficult than in Taiwan. Some of the problems identified with the record keeping system in Indonesia was the frequent rotation of healthcare staff, errors in transferring data from patient records to excel sheets, and data being lost after patients completed treatment (Rachmani, Kurniadi, & Hsu, 2013). The need to create an electronic database of leprosy patients was reiterated as well as the use of an electronic data analysis and reporting system. More initiatives like SMS reminders were implemented in Indonesia to address specific problems like low treatment completion rates. These initiatives brought a significant improvement in these rates (Rachmani et al., 2019).

These examples illustrate the rocky road to applying the benefits of computerised health information systems in the leprosy care sector. It also demonstrates that benefits can be gained if some learning and persistence is applied. In countries where the leprosy burden is less than five thousand cases per year, it may be difficult to justify the investment of developing and maintaining a disease specific electronic health information system.

2.4 Knowledge management and its importance in the healthcare and neglected tropical diseases context

Knowledge Management (KM) is a relatively new field that is becoming increasingly relevant to organizations and institutions as the potential of information technologies increases. There is however still no consensus as to the definition of the term (Girard & Girard, 2015), as the definition of knowledge itself is under debate.

Some of the definitions that illustrate the differences in emphasis would be the following:

"*Knowledge Management is the process of creating, sharing, using and managing the knowledge and information of an organization.*

Knowledge Management is the management process of creating, sharing and using organizational information and knowledge." (Girard & Girard, 2015, p. 14)

"*Knowledge management is the deliberate and systematic coordination of an organization's people, technology, processes, and organizational structure in order to add value through reuse and innovation. This is achieved through the promotion of creating, sharing, and applying knowledge as well as through the feeding of valuable lessons learned and best practices into corporate memory in order to foster continued organizational learning.*" (Ermine, 2010, p. 4)

As the above definitions illustrate, KM includes both aspects of capturing, storing, coding and sharing of information and a growing awareness that knowledge is a valuable commodity that is embedded in an organizations culture and workforce, often in non tangible ways.

Most definitions however agree that even though KM is viewed differently in various academic and practical disciplines, it is not simply about shifting information but about contributing to the organizational objectives and adding value to the system.

As mentioned above, the definition of knowledge itself is very fluid. It is agreed that broadly speaking, knowledge can be seen to include both tacit and explicit knowledge.

"*Knowledge is a more subjective way of knowing, typically based on experiential or individual values, perceptions, and experience.*"(Ermine, 2010, p. 9)

When considering information and communication technologies (ICTs) in a knowledge management context, the question inevitably comes up to try and define how knowledge is different from information, and why it matters? Is knowledge not just stored and categorized information as some of the definitions seem to indicate?

Depending on the perspective from which you look at knowledge it could be seen as a non tangible asset with a business hat on, it could be the functional tools to make an organization work, or it can be seen as application of information in the right time and context to improve outcomes. Probably the best answer would be "all of the above".

It would also be safe to say that there is no magic formula or "one size fits all" approach to knowledge management systems, especially considering this subjective nature of knowledge and the complex relationships between humans that govern sharing and learning.

Knowledge management (KM) can shortly be defined as "doing what is needed to get the most out of knowledge resources" (Becerra-Fernandez & Sabherwal, 2014)

KM is particularly relevant to the health sector. The potential and importance for information technology to improve quality of care is widely recognized (Raghupathi & Umar, 2009).

In the healthcare context, there are many areas where knowledge management do play an important role as summarized by Amori et al., (2016). In particular KM was shown to have the following benefits:

- Medical error reduction
- Improving cooperation and innovations
- Improving quality of care
- Cost reduction
- Improving knowledge organization and organizational learning

In a review of systems research priorities for the strengthening of healthcare systems, the innovative application of knowledge management was seen as one of the key challenges for enhancing the health systems research capacity of health departments (Raymond, 2008). This intuitive link between knowledge management and increases in quality and quantity of research was also indicated by Ceballos, Fangmeyer, Galeano, Juarez, & Cantu-Ortiz, (2017). It was also concluded by Paez-Logreira, Zamora-Musa, & Velez-Zapata, (2016) that without a knowledge management model, the incorporation of new teachers and researchers is more difficult because the lack of guidelines and communication protocols.

In a report from the WHO, the potential and diversity of various information enabled technologies to contribute to learning and training also in a developing context is illustrated (Bollinger, Chang, & Jafari, 2013). It is recommended in the report that "*Ministries of health and health professional organizations must fully embrace e-learning through the establishment of standards and accreditation procedures that facilitate the certification and sharing of training programmes for students and of continuing education initiatives for health-care providers*."(Bollinger et al., 2013, p. 4)

In the African healthcare context with many training gaps as well as high staff turnover, this is an important pointer for the future of knowledge management. Within the NTD care system it is also especially relevant as the diagnosis of Leprosy for instance is still primarily clinical in nature.

Some specific challenges to the application of knowledge management in healthcare were also mentioned by Amori, et al., (2016) that would be relevant to the NTD care system. A high level of awareness of the benefits of KM and a strategy for its implementation is needed which may prove difficult to achieve in a typical hierarchical structure of a health department where the NTD department is often neglected. Another specific challenge that was mentioned was the need for confidentiality and security measures within the knowledge management system. This is also of particular relevance to the NTD care system as some of the CM-NTDs are linked to high levels of stigma and social exclusion for instance leprosy.

When considering the implementation of an electronic system with high technical and skill specifications in a public sector context where these resources are scarce, the question of long-term sustainability needs to be considered. Although great advances have been made in recent years generating the capacity to implement and run systems that makes sense within an industrialized context, these systems do not always have the same "fit" outside of that context. For this reason, it would be prudent to consider aspects related to sustainability in evaluating the design and implementation process of the proposed information system.

Useful for this evaluation, although their study was looking at the importance of knowledge management in the UK construction industry, it highlights the importance of knowledge management for the sustainability of an organization:

"The change in business logic means that there is now a shift from focussing on short-term harvesting of the fruits of success (profitability and increasing shareholder value) to nurturing the roots (building knowledge assets and stakeholder value) for long-term trust, improved governance and sustainability." (Robinson, Anumba, Carrillo, & Al-Ghassani, 2006, p. 7)

Having this long-term perspective is especially relevant for the NTD care sector and especially leprosy care, as there are long incubation periods and slow disease trends over many years, for which a health department needs to maintain perspective. Many health departments, especially also in the leprosy care sector have trouble with sustainability as there is often a high staff turnover and knowledge of leprosy and the longer-term goals are hard to maintain.

According to Robinson, et al. (2006) , having a KM strategy is essential for an organization to put KM principles into practice.

They also went on to develop a KM maturity roadmap where an organization can plot itself to help it understand what still needs to be done and how best to develop its KM implementation strategy. This is also very relevant to the health sector, as KM, if implemented at all, is often implemented in an ad-hoc way without a proper strategy.

Robinson, et al. (2006) identified five stages (STEPS) in the maturity roadmap from start-up to sustainability with some characteristics during each stage. Of particular importance, however, were some key success factors that were also identified by Robinson, et al. (2006) that is worth mentioning as it is likely applicable to the KM efforts in the health sector as well. These key success factors are:

- Need to establish a goal, and develop and align KM strategy to business objectives.
- Provide leadership and resources including management support, staff, and budget.
- Implementation needs to be supported by both IT and non-IT tools.
- Recognition of reform needed to address barriers and to facilitate implementation.
- KM performance measures are required to evaluate KM.

From the above we can conclude that KM has a lot to contribute to the healthcare sector in general and to NTDs in particular. We are also aware however that there are many challenges that need to be taken into account in this particular context, for instance, patient confidentiality and long-term sustainability. The application of knowledge management in organizations takes time to mature and requires purposeful leadership to achieve. Accessible tools are available to measure this maturity and to give guidance even to health departments wanting to embark on this journey.

2.5 The importance of information and communication technology for knowledge management

Information is a key ingredient for all management and decision-making processes. For healthcare systems on various levels this is no exception, especially taking into account the many variables influencing the health outcomes of the healthcare system.

"Health information systems (HIS) are dealing with processing data, information, and knowledge in health care environments." (Winter et al., 2010)

Health information systems have been around before the invention of the computer, and it does not necessarily have to be digitized. In most information systems there are usually a combination of manual, paper based, and electronic tools being used to gather, compile and transfer the information. The information systems in use for the leprosy care system worldwide for instance have been paper based since its inception, and have remained virtually unchanged in may endemic settings.

We are, however, in a context of rapidly expanding mobile and social networks with digital communication technology being ever more prevalent and integrated, even within the rural African context, that it creates possible new opportunities to impact the outcomes of Health Information Systems. Increasingly, health departments around the world and also in Africa are recognizing the importance and potential impact of electronic health information systems to support decision making on various levels (Wager, Lee, & Glaser, 2017). It was assumed that the use of ICT would lead to greater efficiency in the use of resources and have the potential to transform healthcare systems for better service delivery (Shekar, 2012).

Damitew & Gebreyesus (2005) have summarized the advantages of computerized health information systems in comparison to paper-based systems in the following way:

- processing and analyzing large amounts of data quickly
- producing a wide variety of reports from a single data set
- reducing duplication of work
- improving data quality through for example automatic validation during data entry
- improving analysis and presentation, which facilitates interpretation and use.

Other specific benefits that were identified were process efficiency and satisfying information needs.

In a recent review of the benefits of digital health for providers within the British National Health Healthcare system it was found that it improves outcomes, promotes patient independence and shifts the focus to prevention (Deloitte, 2015), all of which is very relevant also for the NTD care system. Most health departments have already installed integrated electronic reporting systems for major diseases and health indicators and some are even experimenting with m-Health tools for data collection for instance the various mHealth initiatives in Kenya and Ethiopia linked to Community volunteers in the HIV care sector, Maternal and child health or e-learning (The World Bank, 2014), (Salte, 2014). In particular the DHIS2 platform has been used in at least 46 countries and is the health information system most commonly adopted within the African context, for instance in Sierra Leone, Ghana, Kenya and Uganda (Dehnavieh, et al., 2018).

A model illustrating the processes in Knowledge Management was developed by Owen & Burstein, (2005) referring to the interconnected processes of Knowledge Capturing, Knowledge Creation, Knowledge Transferring and Knowledge Reusing.

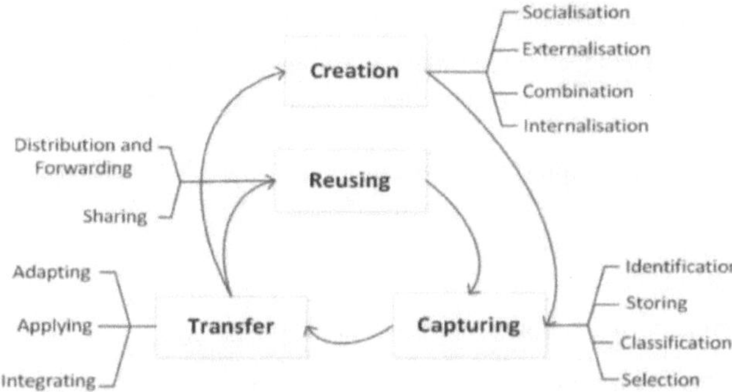

Illustration 1: Framework for KM processes & sub-processes (Owen and Burstein 2005)

Using this model, (Hamad, Wahid Bakar., (2018) concludes that information and communication technologies have become critical enablers for all these processes in knowledge management and is an enabler for organizational change.

Despite the great potential of electronic information systems in general, there have been some very costly failures where man and machine have not come to a satisfactory synergy. According to Lippeveld, Sauerborn, & Bodart (2000) it seems like Health Information Systems in most countries are not managing to deliver on their promises of giving adequate support to management, as they are often data driven and not action driven. Five main reasons for this unfortunate result were the following:

- irrelevance of the information gathered
- poor quality of data
- duplication and waste among parallel health information systems
- lack of timely reporting and feedback
- poor use of information

In evaluating the failure of an extensive Health Information system in South Africa, the evaluation team also added the following factors as reasons for the failure of the system: (Littlejohns, 2003)

- Failure to take into account the social and professional cultures of healthcare organisations and to recognise that education of users and computer staff is an essential precursor

- Underestimation of the complexity of routine clinical and managerial processes
- Dissonance between the expectations of the commissioner, the producer, and the users of the system
- Implementation of systems is often a long process in a sector where managerial change and corporate memory is short
- "My baby" syndrome
- Reluctance to stop putting good money after the project is clear to fail
- Failure of developers to look for and learn lessons from past projects

Introducing health information systems may have many unintended consequences, many of them negative. Coiera, Ash, & Berg, (2016) have for instance illustrated that there are various levels of negative unintended consequences often causing unintended harm to the patient.

From the above, we can conclude that having information and communication systems in use within the healthcare context does not mean that good KM is happening. ICTs within the health system context can be beneficial, but if the bigger goals of the KM system is not understood, the system is likely to fail.

2.6 The importance of the bigger knowledge management goals when introducing information and communication technologies in the healthcare and neglected tropical diseases context

Health Information systems is defined by Lippeveld, Sauerborn, & Bodart (2000, p. 3) as "a set of components and procedures organized with the objective of generating information which will improve health care management decisions at all levels of the health system."
In using this definition we can further break it down by specifically looking at which **components** and which **procedures** would be relevant to make up a health information system in the NTD context.
It is useful to visualize the components of a health information process as set out by Lippeveld, et al., in the following Illustration, as it also shows the relationship between them.

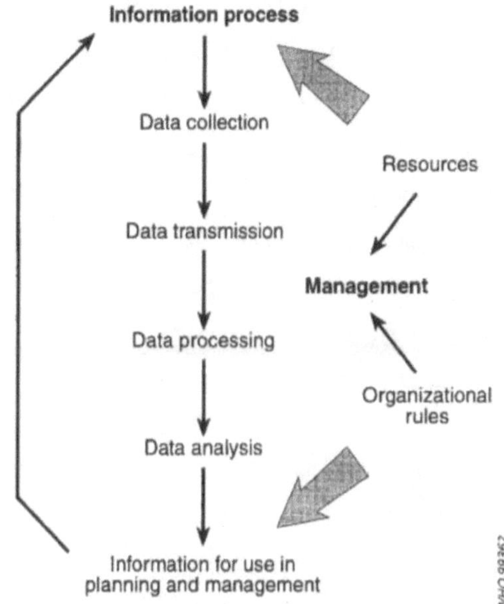

Illustration 2: Components of a health information system (Lippeveld et al., 2000, p. 16)

Of specific relevance is the management components of resources (inputs) and organizational rules and procedures (processes) as major determinants of the use and impact of the information generated by the system. These management components have different complexities depending on the organizational level of the health care system which would define a different set of objectives and stakeholders involved in that level of the care system. These levels are usually defined as primary care, secondary care, and tertiary care. For the purpose of this study we were mainly able to observe the primary level of care in the NTD care system which is at the level of the first patient contact, diagnosis, treatment and case notification. This is mainly due to the greater need at this level, currently, and because the secondary and tertiary care systems are very undeveloped in the Mozambique context so very little data could be gathered here. We were also able to observe the management components in the NTD information system from national level and district level.

Knowing for which level the knowledge management system needs to generate information and decision support, helps to determine the scope and complexity of the components for the health information system to be introduced. The above illustration is of further use as a basis for a conceptual model of a health information system as part of the Soft Systems Methodology process followed in this study.

According to the WHO (2008) and Lippeveld, et al. (2000), a good Health Information System (HIS) has the following key **procedures** or functions, namely **data generation, compilation, analysis and synthesis, and communication and use**. Other issues also highlighted are related to the types of information that different levels of users may need and the availability of this to them in a relevant form. The involvement and linking of relevant partners involved in the healthcare system is also mentioned, and this aspect is likely more relevant on the communication and use side of the equation. Each of these 4 **procedures** individually are likely important for the whole system to be effective, and it is likely that some of these aspects will have differing challenges in different environments, and the solutions chosen may look totally different for those environments.

As an example of the application of these 4 factors in the NTD knowledge management context, one of the NTD partners (ENVISION, n.d.) produced the following illustration :

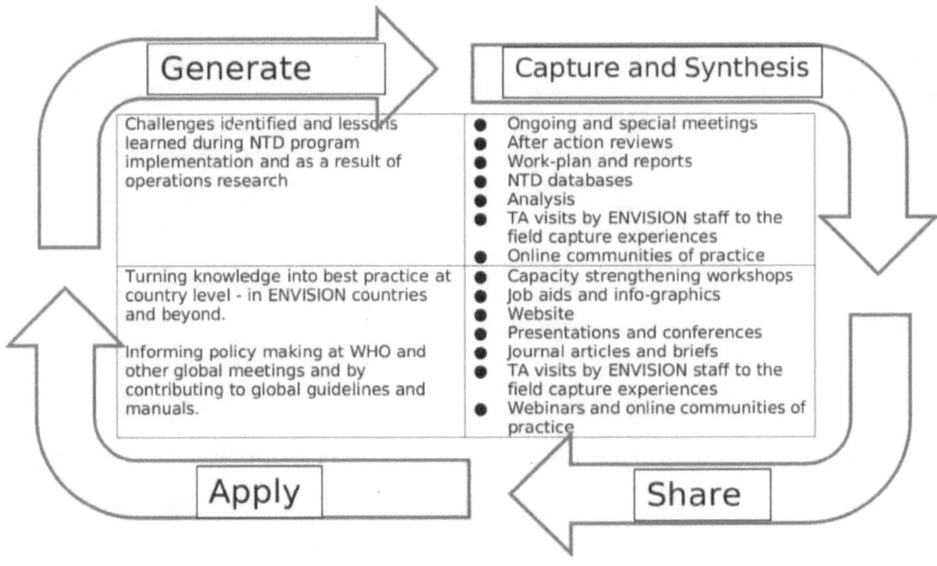

Illustration 3: Systematic knowledge management approach for NTD leadership

(ENVISION, n.d.)

As can be seen from this example, the 4 **functions** of a good Health information system need to work together in a system for knowledge management to have a greater impact, depending of the specific goals set for the system. In the ENVISION example, the goal was to provide global leadership in the NTD care sector. For the CM-NTDs in Mozambique the goal may be improved quality of care, a reduction in morbidity, or greater stability in maintaining the rare skills needed for leprosy diagnosis in the country. Whatever it may be however, this knowledge management goal needs to be defined clearly so that the scope of these procedures can be contextualized to the level of care needed.

As summarized by Lippeveld, et al. (2000, p. 23) "*The design and implementation of an effective and efficient health information system are intimately linked with and have to fit into the organization of the health system for which it generates information.*"

The goals of the KM system within the specific healthcare context, which includes its structure and key actors, needs to be kept in mind when designing a health information system.

During this study it is therefore important to clearly specify the goals for the KM system and to understand the context within which these goals are to be accomplished. The various knowledge management processes to which the health information system will inevitable contribute form an integral part of the success and final usefulness of the system.

2.7 Theories on the adoption of innovations relevant to health information system implementation

Except for the technical and disease specific challenges posed to the implementation of a new health information system, there are many cultural and contextual factors that may have a very powerful influence on the process of integration in the specific context where it is implemented.

In his book on the Diffusion of Innovation, Prof. Everett M. Rogers unpacked a very comprehensive theory on the processes by which individuals evaluate, adopt or reject innovations they perceive as advantageous (Rogers, 2003). This depends greatly on the characteristics of the decision making unit as well as the characteristics of the particular innovation and the environment in which this decision needs to be made. The specific characteristics of the innovation mentioned were relative advantage, compatibility, complexity, trialability and observability. He also showed that innovations

were not adopted by everyone at the same speed, and that five adopter categories exists namely the initial innovators, early adopters, early majority, late majority and the laggards.
The importance of this is that the the population in the different categories had different processes by which they evaluated an innovation and different communication strategies had to be used to reach each of them.
For integrating a new health information system for leprosy in the NTD care sector this clearly has many important lessons and the communication process by which this is rolled out and endorsed by the health department would be an important aspect to contribute to its success. It would be interesting if implementers of the health information system were aware of these adopter categories and could use the dynamic created by the early adopters in the communication and training strategies to help with the adoption process of the other individuals in this very specific target group.

There are also much criticism of the diffusionist way of thinking and it is seen by some as a top down approach and historically linked to a western colonialist mindset (McMaster, 2001).
From the diffusion of innovations camp there is increasing acknowledgment of the value of local knowledge and experience and the role of communities to finding culturally appropriate solutions to their problems. One such example is the concept of Positive Deviance (PD) as an approach to social change that enables communities to discover the local knowledge and wisdom that they already have and to exploit that dynamic to bring about positive behavioral change (Rogers, Singhal, & Quinlan, 2019). It is an approach where the local community is the owner and implementer of the solution and the role of the outside expert is just to facilitate the process.

In the process of integrating a new health information system in the NTD context in Mozambique, we would do well to keep the above criticism in mind and to give space to hear the local voice and to utilize the local knowledge and systems where possible. Local ownership and buy-in is probably going to be critical factors to assure the system gets adopted but also sustained in the long run.

Another theoretical approach to studying communication systems and technology adoption within social systems has been the Actor-Network Theory (ANT). ANT began as a theory mainly in the sociology domain and has also been applied to study communication's role in the constitution of organizations and other phenomena within and around organizations (Bencherki, 2017). Very simplistically put, the theory considers the world to consist of interconnected networks. Actors within these networks can be both human and non-human aspects like machines or projects. Through the convergence of the interests of the heterogeneous actors, networks of interest and association start to grow into conceptual realities called "black boxes" (McMaster, Vidgen, & Wastell, 1997). Each of the actors in the network translates the conceptual reality, for instance a specific innovation, into the specific meaning and purpose that it has for their context and contributes their own resources and thus contributes to shaping the black box for themselves and others. As more actors are enrolled in a network and start to contribute to either validate or adapt the concept, it is strengthened and propagated. The opposite could occur if the actors perceive the meaning or purpose of the conceptual reality (black box) of less value for instance due to a changing environment and start to dissociate from the network and the black box would grow dimmer.

For our implementation of a new information system for the NTD context in Mozambique, this theory has some good learning points. It is important that we enroll all the actors in the system that would be affected by the new innovation and understand their point of view and how the new information system would influence them both positively and negatively. It is also important that we look to how these actors are linked to each other and how they network and interact with each other, as this will also influence the process of translating the new system to their realities or how they may influence that process for each other. If a network of use and affirmation is not built up around the information system, it will not find any sustainable foothold for it to continue in the long run.

Another important aspect to consider is the fact that the conceptual reality (black box) or in our case the health information system, is also changed by the network and the actors. It is important to allow for this and to have the feedback mechanisms within the network and the technical capacity to adapt it locally to be better responsive to the needs and environment of the actors. If this is not done there may be more resistance to its use or it may become irrelevant to the actors over time. This is a real risk as controlling actors within a formal institutional setting like a government health department may not be open to change or to have other actors or users adapt their standardised and controlled instance.

As ANT sees human and non-human entities connected as equals in networks, it has been seen as a very applicable theory for the study of information systems as this also is focused on interaction of humans with technology and information systems. It has been used in various studies to look at network stability and technological adoption and the utility of ANT can be more enhanced if it can be expressed in graphical form (Alexander & Silvis, 2014).
In considering a study methodology or describing the relationships between actors in the neglected tropical diseases care sector in Mozambique, it would be useful if this can be done in some graphical form. This brings to mind the rich pictures used in the soft systems methodology process and the conceptual models developed from it.

In an article on how ANT can be used to study the implementation of information technologies in the healthcare context, Cresswell, Worth, & Sheikh, (2010) noted that ANT can be a tool for sampling by focusing on the different informants that are related to the specific technology that is to be implemented. These informants can be from multiple locations but they are purposefully connected in relation to each other through the technology that is being introduced, which is also seen as an actor. This is likely an important aspect as the neglected tropical diseases care sector is divided across multiple locations and with actors of varying levels of responsibility and training. The perspectives and perceived objectives of the different levels of actors in the NTD care sector may be very different but with the introduction of an information system initiative they are linked to each other in new ways, creating new power balances as the technology is translated from the perspective of each. It is therefore important to sufficiently include actors from various levels of the NTD care sector that these perspectives can be understood and the relationships and networks incorporated.

Many shortcoming of ANT are also mentioned in particular in relation to its use in information system studies as noted by Cresswell et al., (2010):

- The approach is too descriptive and can limit the ability to make concrete suggestions on actors and their behavior.
- ANT is able to describe how things occur, but is weak in giving insights as to why they

occur.

- It is difficult to test with empirical evidence as it is very broad and therefore difficult to verify empirically.

It is therefore suggested to combine other theoretical approaches especially for analysis and interpretation, and to be very focused on the study aims and not get lost in too many details.

2.8 Health information systems implementation and knowledge management in the African and Mozambique contexts

The transfer of technology from a northern to a southern context has its particular challenges. In examining the integration process of health information systems (HIS) in the Mozambique context, Nhampossa (2005) highlighted the following issues to mediate the transfer of technology:

- the need to cultivate the installed base using gradual versus radical change strategies;
- to develop mediating mechanisms to enable participatory processes;
- the need to find a pragmatic balance between internationalization and localization with process rather than product orientation as the underlining objective.

He further argues that the process of "transfer" should rather be seen as a process of "translation" into another context:

"technology is developed as a result of the interaction of culture (manner or way of thinking, talking and acting), context or environment (e.g. country, organization or department), work practices, and the material characteristics of the technology itself. When technology which has been developed within a certain cultural and organizational context is transferred to another, it is confronted with serious socio-technical challenges. To overcome these challenges, this book emphasizes that technology needs to be translated and not just transferred from one context to another."

(Nhampossa, 2005, p. 155)

He then goes on to identify four influences on this translation process, each having multiple points to ponder of their own:

1. history: legacy systems and installed base;
2. the role of adaptation: how software is adapted to the local context;
3. the role of participation: how users exercise control over HIS; and,

4. the process of customization: the balance between localization and internationalization.

The points raised under participation of users in the "translation" process was especially relevant, as it also had implications for the longer-term sustainability of the system in the new context.

Within the Ministry of Health in Mozambique, there is growing experience in utilizing health information systems like DHIS2, for example, in managing healthcare personnel within country. Sustainability remains a concern, however, in the Mozambique context, for instance, to maintain technical staff for the maintenance of the health information systems. To this regard Waters, et al. (2016) made some practical proposals that could be directly relevant to the implementation of a health information system for NTDs in the Mozambique context:

- The extensive intersectoral collaboration between many diverse stakeholders demonstrates their united belief in the viability of the HIS to produce results useful for decision making.
- Conducting a customized assessment of existing systems and procedures prior to system design.
- Utilizing local technical support and building the capacity of the MOH.
- Avoiding the proliferation of multiple partial or geographically focused information systems.
- Continuous process of evolution and development through the dynamic involvement of key stakeholders.

The sustainability of health information systems is further explored by Kimaro & Nhampossa, (2004) who examines aspects of three key relationships during the information system development process, as illustrated in the following diagram taken from their research:

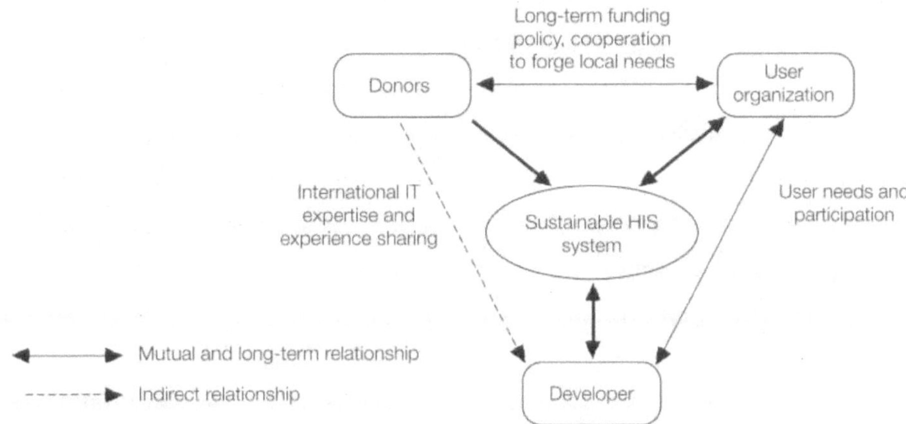

Illustration 4: Network of aligned actors towards a sustainable IT (Kimaro & Nhampossa, 2004, p. 8)

From their analysis, they highlight the long-term vision required to maintain the relationships needed to assure better sustainability of the system to be implemented. This has many direct implications for the development and integration of a system for the NTD department as these projects usually have short-term donors and short contractual relationships with IT developers who may not be available to give longer term support to the process once their contracts come to an end.

In a study reviewing the adoption factors influencing the adoption of information and communication technologies by healthcare professionals it was found that system usefulness and ease of use were the most common ICT adoption facilitators among the study papers reviewed (Gagnon et al., 2012). The study also identified many barriers that would hinder adoption of the ICT which included design and technical concerns, lack of compatibility (with work process, values, etc), time constraints, role boundaries, and lack of perceived usefulness. This gives some pointers to the training priorities for the intended users of the system, as well as for the need to include the end users in the design and implementation processes of the intended system.

Although the above work and especially that of Everett Rogers was done across many cultures and for many different types of innovations, the question still remains if there are specific characteristics within the African or Mozambique contexts that would influence the distribution of adopter categories or the communication objectives for each to enhance the adoption of a health information system for this context. For instance in a study on the importance of trust and risk in the m-commerce sector in South Africa, Joubert & Van Belle, (2009) highlighted the importance of the perceived trustworthiness of the service provider and the legislative environment to enforce correct service delivery or protect the client. These would be important factors in the African context where the best practices and standards are not regularly implemented and the legislative environment is not conducive to protecting the customers.

In an analysis of the factors influencing the adoption of smart phones by Nigerian undergraduate students, it was found by Elogie, Ikenwe, & Idubor, (2015) that the only technological characteristics that explained adoption were relative advantage and complexity. This adoption process was strongly supported by interpersonal communication. Providers of services or technologies should thus not make too many assumptions as to what would motivate the adoption of their innovation in the African context.

Some important lessons can also be learned from a study done on the adoption intention of m-commerce in the Malaysian context among generation X users. Moorthy et al., (2017) found that the literacy level of the users was a direct barrier for the usage of the mobile devices as users were limited to secure their confidential information or the progress of transactions to make a payment. For the African and in particular the Mozambique context this might be very relevant as Mozambique still has a very low literacy rate of just 60% (UNESCO, n.d.) even though it would be assumed that healthcare workers would be at the upper end of the spectrum.

In another example of the adoption of pedagogically-based technology in African higher education contexts, Kizito, (2016) found that a clear strategy for adoption was important to increase chances of successful adoption. This needs to be carried by a supportive infrastructure and a maintenance plan backed by the institution.

As in the study of Gagnon et al., (2012) mentioned above, the time and workload of the participants was also a barrier if it was not considered during the implementation process. An important factor

that was also mentioned was the lack of policy guiding the implementation process indicating a lack of planning and commitment to sustainability.
All these factors would be of great relevance in the Mozambique context where good initiatives often fall prey to these systemic shortcomings.

A recent systematic review of research on the opportunities, barriers, and adoption factors of mobile commerce for the informal sector in developing countries in Africa Pankomera & van Greunen, (2019) gave a very comprehensive overview of factors that may be relevant in this specific context. The following are some of the more relevant adoption categories that were identified by the review :

- **Technical factors** including mobile network coverage and availability of electricity.
- **Awareness or knowledge of adopter**. When a party already has some knowledge of the new technology, the adoption occurs more easily.
- **Perceived usefulness and ease of use**.
- **Affordability or perceived cost**. For instance when normal feature phones can be used to access m-commerce costs are perceived lower and people adopt more.
- **Perceived security and trust**. People perceive mobile platforms to be vulnerable to fraudulent activities online and are concerned about security and confidentiality of personal information.
- **Accessibility**. When m-commerce platforms are designed to target the poor and vulnerable, more people can adopt the platform. Also if it gives access to a broader range of services.
- **Social factors, human capital, and asset endowment**. People are easily influences by the attitudes and behavior of peers. Those with greater access to financial means and assets adopt new technology quicker.

Although this study was focused specifically on m-commerce, many parallels can still be drawn for the adoption factors that would influence the integration of a health information platform in the Mozambique context. For instance the coverage of mobile networks in the various districts of Mozambique, internet connectivity and the experience of the users with mobile phones or a mobile data collecting platform. The training system would need to demonstrate the value that is added for users to use the system and convince them of the ease of use. Security of patient data is of course paramount in relation to leprosy patient data and users would want to know if they would have access to the needed equipment and maintenance for the system to continue to function without creating additional personal costs.

In addition to the adoption factors as identified by this study, a number of barriers were also highlighted. These include financial, technical, social, and cultural barriers. A particular barrier that was mentioned was high levels of illiteracy in certain African countries that hindered m-commerce adoption. While we would expect healthcare workers needing to interact with a health information system to be literate, the same can likely not be said for many community healthcare workers that are some of the main sources of patient information for the leprosy supervisors. As Mozambique is a Portuguese speaking country, care should be taken to adequately translate the interface.

Closer to the Mozambique context and in a completely non ICT field, the adoption decision to use fertilizers for small scale agriculture by rural Mozambican farmers were the subject of a randomised study. This study evaluated the impact of a one time voucher for fertilizer and better seeds, but also evaluated the persistence of impacts on the household fertilizer use and economic status in subsequent years (Carter, Yang, & Laajaj, 2014). There was considerate persistence of impacts on fertilizer usage and also household outcomes up to three years after the one time subsidy was given. This was directly related to the individual learning via their own experience or the experience of others in their social network that received the vouchers. The expectations of better returns from using fertilizer was raised by being allotted a voucher, but fertilizer use was especially strongly influenced by the number of voucher winners in the social network of participants.

Even though this example may not be related to the adoption of information and communication technology, it still hints to the importance of creating positive expectations for an adoption decision and also to the importance of shared learning within social networks in Mozambique. The experiences of other healthcare workers in engaging with the proposed health information platform will have a strong influence on the decision to adopt it or not. Opportunities for shared group learning might be an important tool in the roll-out or training processes.

In another study on the dynamics of adoption and use of ICT based initiatives in the Mozambique context, the argument is made by Macome, (2002) that the theory of diffusion of innovations as set out by Everett Rogers makes many assumptions on the homogeneity of the institutional environment where innovations are adopted as well as the invariable nature of innovations over time as they pass through sequential stages. It is suggested by Macome, (2002) that the Actor-Network Theory may be a way of overcoming some of the limitations of the diffusion theory and may be more appropriate for the Mozambique context. Macome then goes on to consider the four obligatory passage points (OPP) of translation that an innovation could pass through as described by Callon, (1984). These passage points are :

- The **problematisation** or how to become an indispensable actor
- The devices of '**interessement**' or how the allies are locked into place
- **Enrolment**: How to define and co-ordinate the roles
- The **mobilisation** of allies: the spokespersons as representative

The findings of this study in the Mozambique context suggest that integration of ICT related initiatives are better when the initiative is integrated with the core productive actions or objectives of the organization. The study also identified other initiatives that improved institutionalization of ICT initiatives like consultations, debate and negotiations among the actors.
For the integration of the health information system in the NTD context in Mozambique, these are very valuable points of advice. The main implementing institution, which is the NTD sector within the health department, needs to take strong ownership of the initiative and should have a strong understanding how the information system could add value to their core purpose. The importance of mobilizing the local interest and support of the larger group of actors is again highlighted. Ways should be sought to increase awareness, receive feedback and stimulate engagement among these key actors to increase their connection to the ICT initiative during the roll-out process.

In conclusion we now have some perspective on the specific neglected tropical diseases context and in particular of leprosy. As one of the older and slower progressing neglected tropical diseases, leprosy needs a long term perspective as well as credible data in order to track disease trends and possibly attract investment to fight the disease. Even though the disease specific indicators for leprosy have a high level of standardisation between most countries, there have been few successful examples of moving the country leprosy records to an electronic format, or to collect case data electronically. This is a big hindrance to disease control program development and a lost opportunity for leprosy epidemiological research.

From the examples of previous information system deployments in the NTD and particularly the leprosy care sector, we are aware that more are at stake than just the roll-out of data gathering tools. The concept of knowledge management is introduced and the specific relevance of this is emphasised for the NTD and leprosy care sectors. A sustainable objectives focused care system is needed that knowledge contributes to, and not simply the gathering of data. The importance of clearly defining knowledge management goals for the care system context where the health information system will be implemented, is also emphasised. This context includes its structure and key actors that needs to be kept in mind when designing a health information system.

For the design of this study the implication is that we need to define the system under scrutiny within the NTD levels of care very clearly. This will further help us determine the objectives of the actors within that level of care which will help define the objectives of the knowledge management initiative we are trying to introduce. The relationships between various levels of care would also need to be demonstrated.

Except for the technical and disease specific challenges in implementing a new health information system, there are many cultural and contextual factors that would influence the outcomes of this venture. A few theoretical models for integrating new innovations are considered and it is clear that from a theoretical perspective at least, there are many important relevant lessons to be learned for the NTD care system in Mozambique. These theoretical perspectives also provide some useful pointers for the design of this study for instance to use graphical representations of actor networks where possible. It is also suggested to select as wide a network of actors as possible even if they are geographically distant from each other. A strong focus on the study objectives is advised for the analysis of data so that useful conclusions can be made.

Specifically from an African and even Mozambique context, we see however that the specific

characteristics of the actors needs to be kept in mind. Aspects like illiteracy, different communication channels, social networks, previous exposure to similar systems and learning styles would strongly influence the process of adoption in this context.
The study should therefore try to understand the relevant actors better and also try and measure the level of expose of the selected participants to similar technologies.

Many institutional and economical factors, as mentioned by various researchers from the African and Mozambique perspectives, are also considered and links made to the NTD care context. Of specific relevance for this study would be to understand the institutional actor who would be considered as the owner of the NTD care system under study. The objectives of this actor would have direct bearing on the objectives of the knowledge management initiative and long term sustainability as well.

3 Research Methodology.

3.1 Study design and study population

As we have seen from the literature review above, the introduction of a KM system would require an analysis of the specific context, including historical factors, cultural factors, and interlinked relationships between actors within the system. It would also have to be able to give some guidance in evaluating the objectives for the knowledge management system as this is essential for the design and implementation of the system. As this study was done during the process of designing and implementing a health information system for the Mozambique NTD sector, it was not possible to remain outside of the situation as a neutral observer. The author was part of the implementation team and lessons learned or new perspectives were fed back into the design and implementation process. This being the case, it seemed appropriate to use some form of action research methodology.

Action Research is a methodology that involves actively participating in a situation that you want to change, going through cycles of reflection and learning, and solving problems in a participatory way. Action research has been used in a variety of fields to do research and solve practical problems, and the approach has been adapted by various researchers and practitioners for specific settings. One such adaptation is Soft Systems Methodology (SSM) developed by Peter Checkland and Brian Wilson, "who through "action research" were able to put together a practical and pragmatic approach to the identification and solution of "soft" ill-defined problems" (Burge, 2015, p. 1).
SSM is based on Systems Theory, which is evident from its methodology that alternates between looking at real world situations and then creating structured systems definitions which ultimately "*produces a set of feasible and culturally-acceptable actions which can be taken to improve the problem situation*" (Gasson & Group, 1994, p. 1).

The usefulness of SSM in the development of information systems has been well established and seems particularly relevant where "the problem situation is seen as "fuzzy" or ill-defined. In other words, it is not immediately clear what type of system or systems will solve the problems of the organisational work-system" (Gasson & Group, 1994, p. 2)

This description seems to fit the Mozambique context well where there is no clear indication as to the best way forward in implementing a health information system for the NTD department, and where there is also little evidence that this will contribute to improve KM as we would like to see.

"The major advantage of applying the SSM to KM research is that it includes explicit modelling of the context of the research, which is absolutely essential to when talking about knowledge as opposed to information management" (Fennessy, Gabby & Burstein, 2000, p. 181).

From an Actor-Network theory (ANT) perspective, soft systems thinking encourages multiple perspectives on an issue or an innovation (McMaster, 2001) in that it helps us understand better how actors are linked to each other in their network and where a new innovation would fit in and influence the system.

Involving the researcher and the users more actively might possibly have other unintended but hopefully beneficial results as argued by Harrison and Zappen "Not only should researchers be involved in ICT design and development, but they should invite and integrate the perspectives of users for whom ICTs are designed and delivered. When this is done, it becomes possible to create technology systems that serve a different set of social needs and interests, in this case, those related to the enhancement of democracy and community." (Harrison & Zappen, 2003, p 21)

SSM in its original form has seven stages in its inquiry process. The process can start at any stage and can move forwards or backwards as the situation requires, or as new insights or perspectives comes to light during the process. It typically has a cyclic nature where outputs may start new cycles of the process, with the aim of leading to change or an improvement of the situation.

"SSM is a facilitative method for organisational investigation: the investigator does not model the "system" in isolation, but facilitates (provides support for) organisational actors in their modelling of the organisational "system"" (Gasson & Group, 1994, p. 2)

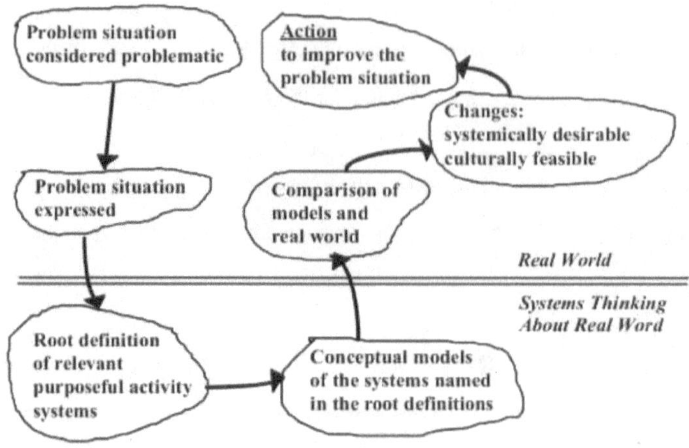

Illustration 5: The seven stages of a Soft Systems Methodology process

The seven stages of the SSM inquiry are the following:

1. The problem situation unstructured: At this stage of the process as many possible different views and perspectives from actors are sought, even though it may seems bit messy and unstructured.
2. The problem situation expressed: The facilitator in conjunction with actors attempt to express the situation in the form of a drawing or some graphical representation. As many varied perspectives are incorporated as possible to show their relationship.
3. Root definitions of relevant systems: Following a systematic arrangement of actors and processes derived from a CATWOE analysis, the purpose of the system under study is defined.
4. Deriving conceptual models: Using the root definition as a basis, the conceptual model is a representation of how such a system and purpose can be achieved under ideal circumstances.
5. Comparing conceptual models with the real world: The ideal and the reality is compared and lessons are learned on how the current system can maybe be adapted for where bottlenecks can be resolved.
6. Defining feasible, desirable changes: Lessons are captured and priorities are set to improve the functioning of the system.
7. Taking action: The above is implemented.

The process looks at the real-world situation as it is, in as much detail as possible including the world views of the actors involved and a wider analysis of issues relevant to the system. The CATWOE analysis leads the participants to define the basic components of a working system which are summed up with the acronym CATWOE:

C - Customers who (or what) benefits from this transformation

A - Actors who facilitates the transformation to these customers

T - Transformation from “start” to “finish”. What the system changes or produces.

W - Weltanschauung what gives the transformation some meaning. Why do we do it ?

O - Owner to whom the “system” is answerable and/or could cause it not to exist

E - Environment that influences but does not control the system

Using the root definition, the process then builds system models of the world as it might be or should be following a structured process, and then compares the real world and systems models with each other. Comparing these models leads to debate and learning (research) as well as actions to improve the situation.

3.2 The study population and sampling technique

For an action research-based study like SSM a qualitative based methodology is likely to be a more practical approach as most of the data / information would be unstructured and un-quantifiable. A qualitative study also allows for the study of issues in more depth and allows for more detail to be included (Patton, 2015). The systematic and structured approach of SSM builds on the strengths of qualitative inquiry which is particularly oriented towards exploration and inductive logic (Patton, 2015).

As the aim of this study was not to make generalized conclusions but to get a greater perspective within this specific context, a **nonprobability sampling** technique was used. Using a nonprobability technique implies that subjective methods are used to determine the selection of elements to be included in the study. (Millet, 2009).

As part of the SSM process that was followed, some specific groups and individuals were selected on the basis of their knowledge and experience in the NTD care environment and as users of the proposed knowledge management system. For this reason the specific sampling technique used in this study was **judgmental / purposive sampling** as defined by Robinson

Purposive sampling is intentional selection of informants based on their ability to elucidate a specific theme, concept, or phenomenon." (Robinson, 2014)

As stated previously, the author was closely involved in the design and implementation of the study. There is clearly the possibility that the sampling or findings can be influenced or biased in some way by this involvement, but it is hoped that the involvement contributed to a greater depth and perspective as stated by Patton "...closeness does not make bias or loss of perspective inevitable; distance is no guarantee of objectivity." *(Patton, 2015, p. 49)*

From a systems theory perspective, the system under study was defined as the following:

"The CM-NTD care system"

Case Managed Neglected Tropical Diseases (CM-NTDs) is a subgroup of NTDs, falling under the NTD department of the Ministry of Health. The National Leprosy Program also falls under the NTD department and has a dedicated national coordinator.

On provincial level, there is a Provincial NTD supervisor in each province overseeing all of the NTDs.

In each district there are NTD district supervisors who usually also double as the tuberculosis supervisor for the district except in a few provinces like Cabo Delgado where they only focus on leprosy and other NTDs. The provincial and district supervisors are responsible to implement the national NTD and leprosy control plans within each province. For leprosy in particular, this includes diagnosing and notifying of new cases and following up on treatment until the end of the treatment cycle.

The leprosy program relies heavily on trained community healthcare volunteers in many villages to identify possible new cases of leprosy, refer them to the health services, and in the case of diagnosis to coordinate the treatment at a community level.

Other health-care services occasionally involved in the care system would be health-post nurses and rehabilitation services to manage complications caused by the diseases.

The proposed new health information system for this NTD care sector is based on a DHIS2 server hosted and maintained by the National ministry of health. This system should be integrated into the existing national DHIS2 health information infrastructure. Data collection principally occurs on the level of the District supervisors who was equipped with an Android based tablet with a DHIS2 mobile application installed for the data gathering of newly diagnosed cases. Data is synchronized to the central DHIS2 framework via a mobile internet connection or any Wifi connections on district or provincial level. District and Provincial supervisors have access to a dashboard either on the DHIS mobile application or on a web browser where data can be verified and indicators tracked.

In summary, the actors within this system (and its sub-systems) were the following groups and institutions:

	Group or institution	Approximate number of people/units in this subsystem	Number of participants in study and level of participation.
1	Undiagnosed patients	Due to the long incubation time, it is not possible to have an accurate estimate.	N/A
2	Diagnosed patients (leprosy, LF and trachoma trichiasis)	+- 1100 new patients (leprosy) per year. LF and trichiasis without records.	This group was not interviewed as they were not directly linked to the proposed health information system.
3	NTD Village health volunteers	+- 1750 in the country	This group was not interviewed as they were not directly linked to the proposed health information system.
4	Selfcare groups	+- 120 groups in the country	This group was not interviewed as they were not directly linked to the proposed health information system.
5	NTD contact Health post nurses	1067 (Lindelöw, Ward, & Zorzi, 2004)	This group was not interviewed as they were not directly linked to the proposed health information system. Perspectives was gathered through the District Supervisor engagements.

6	District Supervisors	160	Convergent interviews : 4 Group discussions : 160 participants during the roll out process in each province.
7	Provincial Supervisors	11	Convergent interview : 3 Group discussions – 11 participants during the roll out process along with district supervisors. User feedback review – 11
8	National Leprosy Coordinator	1	Convergent interview : 1 Group discussions : was present during the roll out process and discussions in most provinces.
9	National NTD program staff	3	Individual interview : 1
10	National health information system management team.	2	Participated in group discussions during the planning and pilot review meetings.

Table 1: Actors in the NTD care sector

For the integration of a Health information system the participant groups 6-10 (see above table) would be the primary contributors and users of the proposed health information system being introduced by the NTD department. The study managed to engage with most of them in some way or another either through individual interviews or during the initial development of "Rich Pictures" and conceptual models, or in subsequent cycles of the action research process as users of the information system.

Groups 1-5 are not directly linked to the proposed health information system, but they are key players in the CM-NTD care system. Subsequent KM processes flowing from the use of the proposed health information system would lead to their involvement and contribution to knowledge within the system. The initial intention was to include these groups also in individual interviews, but this was not practically possible at the time. It was decided to limit the scope of the study and put greater emphasis on the HIS integration process and the knowledge management aspects related to the actors in groups 6-10.

3.3 Data Collection

In following the SSM approach, the aim was to get as good as possible an understanding of the human activity system involved and to give as many actors as possible the opportunity to express their perceptions of the situation.

"To accurately define a problem, it must not come from one person, but must be a shared view."(Seagriff & Lord, 2011, p. 42)

For this reason, the study relied heavily on convergent interviews and facilitated group discussions in order to get a shared view on the NTD care system. The opportunities for these facilitated group discussions were also closely linked to the development and implementation process that was followed for the new NTD information system in Mozambique, for instance planning meetings, feedback sessions and evaluation reports. Other data included document analysis of project and planning documents and observations during the project implementation process.

The implementation process had an initial **planning stage** which involved a 3 day inception workshop with a wide selection of stakeholders as well as specific planning meetings with various task teams over a three month period. Two provinces were then selected for the **pilot stage** of the implementation process. A national team was sent to these provinces and all district and provincial supervisors of these two provinces were involved in a 3 to 4 day initiation workshop. After the pilot phase which lasted about a month, a **review** was done of the results and discussed during a review meeting. The information system and implementation methodologies were improved and adapted with each iteration of the implementation in subsequent provinces over the following 9 months. After this **implementation phase** a feedback meeting was held with all the provincial supervisors and national NTD staff where the results were discussed.

The research question and consequential data needs were further unpacked in the following matrix to illustrate where the data collection methods fit in:
Research Question: "What **factors would contribute** to the successful **integration** of a health information system for CM-NTDs in order to **improve Knowledge Management** within the wider NTD care system?"

Research Question element	Type of data needed	Data collection methods used.
"Integrate"	A better understanding of the system context including the key stakeholders and their characteristics.	Observations of NTD care staff in their work environment Convergent interviews with stakeholders. Group discussions and meetings. Document analysis including case registers and reports from districts and provinces.
Factors to Integrate a Health Information system	Factors related to the information system: **Hard factors** would include: • Communication channels • Types of mobile technology available. • User tool characteristics	Communication survey Analysis of current information systems Convergent interviews with stakeholders. Group discussions and

	(mobile apps and Web interface etc.) **Soft factors** would include: • Relationships between actors • Authority structures • Attitudes • Worldview • Etc.	meetings. Rich Pictures
Improved KM in NTDs	Performance Indicators or a framework to evaluate KM performance in this context.	Health Information system database queries. Observations of NTD care staff in their work environment Document analysis including registers and meeting reports

Table 2: Breakdown of the research question

The following data collection methodology was followed:

1. Soft Systems Methodology – Rich picture

To get a better understanding of the current reality within the NTD care system, the major stakeholders were asked to draw a picture (**Rich Picture**) of how they saw the NTD care system. This happened at an inception workshop at the start of the project and had a good representation from all the provinces and many government departments. The picture was drawn in a collective manner during a plenary session, was then discussed and more detail was added during the discussion to clarify interactions between actors, conflicts or specific issues raised. During interviews with District and Provincial supervisors, they were also asked to draw a picture of how they saw their system, giving some more background information to the broader rich picture made during the initial inception workshop.

2. Individual interviews

Interviews with various stakeholders were usually done after program meetings but also during field visits in other provinces. Participants were selected based on their experience and knowledge in the NTD care sector. There is a high staff turnover especially among district supervisors, which limited the choice of people for an interview. Interviews usually lasted between 20-30 minutes and a basic systems framework was used to give an initial structure to the conversation. The framework gave participants the opportunity to express what they saw as their main purpose, why they felt it was important and which resources, actors or other factors made their work easier or more difficult. If any specific positive or negative points were raised, these were then explored further. The interviews were recorded in Portuguese and afterwards transcribed directly into the systems framework according to the themes of Resources, Actors, Activities, Objectives/transformation and Effects. Participants were also asked to draw a picture of their work system and how they relate to actors within the system. Many participants found it difficult to make a graphical representation of their work system. In total 7 individual interviews with supervisors were recorded.

3. Group discussions

Group discussions were held with various stakeholder groups during the course of the project implementation. Some of the discussions were of a more structured nature and were captured in rich pictures or diagrams made jointly by the group, some were recorded, and others were captured by someone taking official minutes of the meeting. Other discussions were of a more informal nature where it was not possible to capture the discussion in a structured way. These informal discussions were however an essential part of the overall SSM process where learning was discussed, changes were made, and new initiatives tested as in an action learning cycle. During the more formal **group discussions**, the conversation was recorded and later transcribed directly into a systems framework. In each of the provinces where the project was implemented, an inception workshop was held with all of the district supervisors as well as the provincial supervisor of that province. During the course of the 3 to 4 days of this workshop there were opportunities where the objectives of the proposed information system were discussed and feedback was received from the users on how they experienced the system, their fears, concerns and realities. This feedback was mostly captured in changes in methodology, system improvements or sometimes a report with recommendations.

4. Documentation and report analysis

During many of the program meetings or project rollouts in various provinces, the participants reported on their situation in the province or district. These reports were collected where possible. Minutes were also taken during some of the meetings and information from these meetings also gave insight into the background situation and some of the learning acquired during the process.

5. Health information system database queries.

Health information statistics on leprosy and other NTD notifications and indicators were also available and gave some insight into the background situation at the time of the study, and also on some of the changes brought about by the new information system that was introduced.

6. Observations from the field

During system roll-out workshops and district, health post and village visits the NTD care system was also observed. Feedback was mostly captured in visit reports or in project planning documents. As in an action research cycle, data gathering did not only happen at the start of the study, but also as feedback was received from stakeholders during the development, piloting, and implementation phases of the project, for instance, as national level data analysts received feedback on the use (or not) of the new system by supervisors after the implementation in different provinces. This data was mostly captured in project reports and planning documents.

7. Expert opinions

The opportunity presented itself during a regional training workshop to learn from others implementing similar systems in other countries. Interviews were done with project developers from Zimbabwe and Ghana that have already implemented similar DHIS2 systems successfully, even though it was not in the NTD sector.

3.4 Data analysis

Soft Systems Methodology (SSM) process

During the SSM action research cycle, qualitative data gathering, and analysis happens in close proximity to each other. The validity of data gathered during individual interviews are also verified during group discussions with different stakeholders. The cyclic nature of the action research process implies that early interpretations can be challenged and refined (Dick & Swepson, 1994).

Dialectics is about creating the opportunity for different points of view to be constructively played of against each other in order to try and come to a better solution or to original approaches (Coccia, 2018), (Spranzi, 2014), (Frauenberger, Foth, & Fitzpatrick, 2018).
A dialectical approach would then try to create such an environment where different opinions are encouraged and different actors encouraged to express them. As a SSM approach tries to bring out different points of view at work within a system where various actors may have competing interests.

For the purpose of this study a 4-stage dialectic approach to SSM, as suggested by Bob Dick (2002) was used. This structure was chosen as it also roughly corresponded to the phases of the implementation process followed for the development and implementation of the information system in Mozambique. During each stage the input from the main actors are sought to help think through the tention situations created for instance between what is (Rich picture) and what should be (Root definition) or between what it should be (Root definition) and what it can be (conceptual models). The process can be summarized in the following diagram:

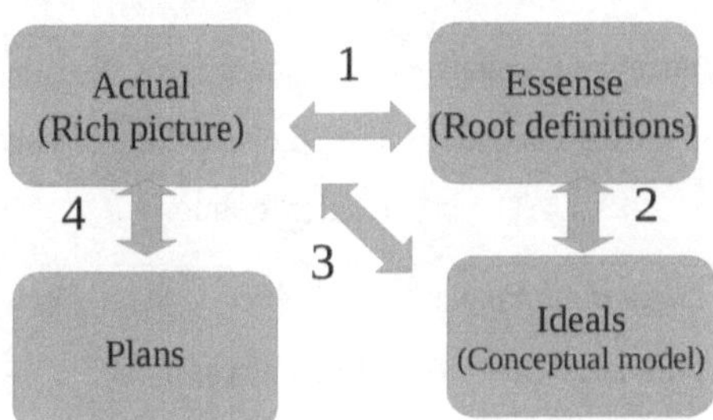

Illustration 6: 4 stage dialectic approach to SSM used during the study

1. The first dialectic between immersion (the rich picture) and essence (the root definitions)
2. The second dialectic between the essence (the root definitions) and the ideals (the conceptual models)
3. The third dialectic between ideals (conceptual models) and reality
4. The fourth dialectic between plans and implementation

The following matrix sets out the data gathering and qualitative data analysis that was used during each of these dialectic stages in the SSM process.

Stage	Main purpose (Why ?)	Data collection methods	Data analysis methods
1. Actual	Understand the context well and build a "Rich Picture" of the situation as well as Root definitions	Convergent interviews with stakeholders. Focus group discussions. HIS database queries.	Rich Picture building CATWOE analysis
2. Essence	Develop Conceptual models and verify the validity of the models.	Convergent Interviews	Input-Output diagrams Root definition creation Conceptual model development
3. Ideals	Compare the conceptual models with reality and identify action points.	Facilitated focus group discussions Expert opinions	Consolidated opinions from stakeholders
4. Plans	Prioritize and create action plans and monitoring framework.	Facilitated focus group discussions	Activity grid.

Table 3: Summary of data gathering and analysis during the SSM process

As mentioned above, data gathering and analysis during the SSM process happened in 4 dialectic engagements:

1. Actual

   During the initial inception workshop and also during interviews with supervisors, **rich pictures** were used as an expression of how the actors saw the system functioning and attaining its goals. As mentioned above, data gathering, and analysis cannot be completely separated during an action research methodology. In drawing the rich pictures along with stakeholders, a lot of discussion and analysis was actually already happening.

In making and discussing the rich pictures some specific issues were already brought to light, for instance, frustrations or conflict points and bottlenecks in the system.

To better understand the perspective at national level, group discussions were facilitated with national level NTD data analysts and the NTD program leadership, sometimes in a more formal structured way, but often in very informal discussions over coffee . **Group discussions** that occurred during various phases of the research, whether in a formal or informal way, also served in analyzing the actual situation. Issues of the current situation were discussed with stakeholders as they became aware of issues raised during the course of the SSM or health system implementation process.

Further background information was gained from the **NTD disease statistics** that were analyzed by the NTD department in producing standard WHO defined disease indicators, following standard protocols. These gave a perspective of current trends and specific epidemiological issues affecting the NTD care system in general and Mozambique specifically. This was further reinforced by **project reports** from many districts and provinces.

At the initiation workshop where the first more comprehensive rich picture was drawn, the first basic **CATWOE analysis** was also done. As individual interviews were done with supervisors and other stakeholders the validity of this analysis was also tested as participants described their objectives, activities and actors from their specific perspectives.

2. Essence

During this phase the emphasis was strongly on analyzing the rich pictures and background data received from interviews and observations. The CATWOE analysis from the previous phase was principally used to develop **input-output diagrams** describing the main transformation intended by the system. Here it became clear that different outcomes were expected from the perspectives of the various stakeholders in the system and that a good balance needed to be found to define what the system actually intended to achieve, and which level of perspective should take precedence.

At a stakeholder meeting after the pilot studies, the root definition was tested and two sets of root definitions were then developed. These root definitions formed the basis of the process to follow, but they were not cast in stone and further reflections followed, especially as more experience was gained from the roll-out and development of the system in other provinces.

The results of the various interviews were compared and common themes were identified and grouped using a basic systems structure:

Resources/Input > Activities [In the context of: Background/Conflict/Vision] > Why - Transformation and Weltanschhaung

A separate consolidated summary was made for the District Supervisors and the Provincial Supervisors as their perspectives on their system could be very different. The objective was not primarily to make a statistical analysis of the themes that came out, but to gain more background information on the leprosy/NTD care system, identify conflict points, and verify the rich picture that had been developed. This feedback was then summarized in a consolidated systems framework for both the District and Provincial supervisors separately.

3. Ideals

The objective during this phase was to formulate a better perspective of how the system should operate within a system-thinking perspective. The understanding gained from the root definition and other input was used to find opportunities to engage with stakeholders and find ways to move closer to the ideal.

To formulate a proposal of a more ideal system, the root definitions of the previous steps were used to formulate a conceptual model. This model tries to visually summarize the most ideal way to achieve the desired transformation from a system thinking perspective. Another very useful way to gain a new perspective and to verify the conceptual models was to gain some outside input from other countries that are also implementing similar health information systems within Africa.

As part of the action research process, there were many opportunities for engagement with stakeholders, especially during the iterative process of implementing the health information system in the various provinces of Mozambique. There were also various opportunities to analyze the results of the previous implementations in provinces along with key stakeholders and to adapt the system or the implementation process for the next provincial implementation. This happened during feedback meetings after the pilot study and planning meetings with the health ministry and the system developers.

4. Plans

   During the action research cycle there were two main groups of lessons learned.

   One group that flowed especially from the many iterations during the implementation in the provinces. This group of lessons was about the procedures that was followed for the system to be implemented.

   The other group of learning was more from the SSM process and consisted of indications from a wider systems perspective on what needs to be done for the system to better achieve its goals as a health information system pointing to knowledge management.

   To provide stronger links to the ultimate goal of improving knowledge management within the NTD care system, the knowledge management performance measurement framework adapted by Faisst & Resatsch (2004) was used as a framework to cast the results and conclusions into where possible:

<table>
<tr>
<td><u>Cost indicators (Class II)</u>
Costs of interventions
Interceding processes.
Encompasses the costs of running the Knowledge management system. <u>What effort is needed to keep it going?</u></td>
<td><u>Intermediation and transfer indicators (Class III)</u>
System usage
User satisfaction
Knowledge transfer within the organization.
<u>Is the right knowledge getting to the right places / users ?</u></td>
<td><u>Effect indicators on business results (Class IV)</u>
Business results (Health service outcomes)
<u>Is the knowledge changing anything for the better ?</u></td>
</tr>
<tr>
<td colspan="3"><u>Knowledge base indicators (Class I)</u>
System quality, Knowledge quality (Documents), Knowledge specific service.
This encompasses the <u>systems and infrastructure</u> to capture data and knowledge, to organise and store it.</td>
</tr>
</table>

Table 4: Knowledge management performance framework adapted by (Faisst & Resatsch, 2004)

This framework breaks the performance of a knowledge management system into four parts namely

- Knowledge base (quality)
- Cost and sustainability
- Knowledge transfer
- Effect / Impact

This structure was a useful way to consolidate a wide range of learning and also to highlight some key themes in knowledge management that require specific attention. The results was ultimately grouped and prioritized to highlight the essence of the findings and was presented to the health ministry for their evaluation and further action.

3.5 Limitations of the study

As stated above, the author was closely involved in the design and roll out process of the health information system implementation project. To some extent this could have influenced the persons interviewed to either respond according to what they think the author wants to hear, or to withhold some information that could put them in a bad light.

A close personal involvement could also create the possibility of bias towards a good outcome of the project and to ignore negative feedback and outcomes. As this was not a project evaluation and the outcomes of the project was not in play, it is hoped that this would not be the case.

As part of an action research approach, there were plenty of group work and reflection which would hopefully limit the influence of the author and contribute to having a balanced view of the real situation in the NTD care sector.

The sampling of especially the district and provincial supervisors for personal interviews were limited to those that had sufficient knowledge and experience in the NTD care sector. There is a high turnover of healthcare staff, and the objective was to form a balanced view of the functioning of the care sector. For that reason supervisors were not selected randomly, but rather according to their experience in the NTD sector. Time was also limited as interviews had to be done within the process of rolling out the information system in the 2-3 days that there was an opportunity to have contact with supervisors from that particular province. The voice of most supervisors were however heard during the group discussions and the rich picture creation during the initiation workshop.

Apart from the structured interviews, the data gathering was very unstructured and difficult to formalise. Some of the provinces had official reports, but many did not or had a version that was not signed and stamped by district or provincial authorities. A lot of the data came from project planning meetings and was captured in summary reports but not minuted and approved by the same group. Although the soft systems methodology process gives some structure and process to the action research approach, it is recognised that it is difficult to verify data and maintain objective rigor.

Data was of a qualitative nature from a wide spectrum of sources. To try and maintain the focus on the objectives of the study, a knowledge management performance framework was used where possible to help analyse and structure the data. In some cases the data did not speak naturally into this structure and it was structured in other more appropriate ways.

4 Results

4.1 The neglected tropical diseases health information system within the context of the general health information system in Mozambique

"Mozambique's health information systems include a variety of population-based and health facility-based data sources. The main population-based sources of health information are census, household surveys and registration systems. The main health facility-related data sources are public health surveillance, health services data and health system monitoring data including human resources, health infrastructure, and financing." ("Health information system - WHO | Regional Office for Africa," n.d.)

The following diagram borrowed from an assessment of the routine primary care health information system in Mozambique (Gimbel et al., 2011) shows the structure and flow of the health information system data within Mozambique.

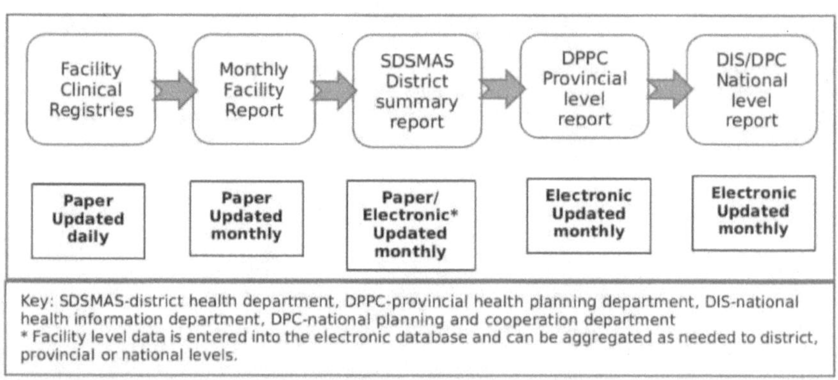

Illustration 7: Mozambique health information data flow diagram

Of note is that the data gets aggregated at the district level and sent to the provincial and national levels in electronic format. This currently happens by means of the DHIS2 system, which has been adopted and rolled out by the health department over the past 6-7 years. Each district has DHIS2 data technicians that receive information in paper format from facilities, in a standardized format according to predefined indicator and data sets. This technician then aggregates the data and inputs it into the DHIS2 database online.

The NTD sector does not, unfortunately, feed into the integrated HIS, and the flow of data is handled in a vertical way. Although national prevalence surveys and mapping have been done for most of the MDA-related NTDs, it was in the form of isolated vertical surveys by donors to follow up on treatment coverage and MDA results.

The Leprosy program and the leprosy information system was also a stand-alone vertical system. At the time this study was initiated, the Leprosy patient registers were paper based with a separate register being kept in each endemic district. For the NTD program manager at national level to have a picture of the situation, they had to gather information from more than 150 book registers from across the country. Apart from Leprosy, none of the other CM-NTDs in Mozambique had any form of regular structured health information gathering.

Typically, the flow of information for the Leprosy program could be summarized in the following diagram:

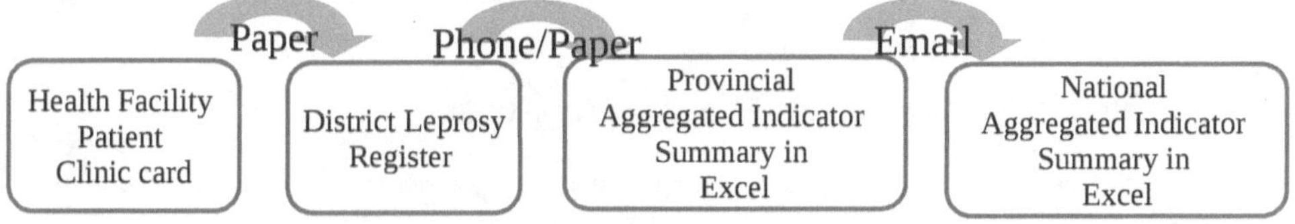

Illustration 8: Information flow in the Leprosy information system in Mozambique

Fortunately, there is a growing awareness of the importance of relevant health information in the Mozambique health department, and currently **the NTD department is undertaking to introduce an electronic case notification system for the Case Managed NTDs (CM-NTDs) in the whole country**.

This would be a third attempt to introduce an electronic notification system for leprosy in Mozambique. A previous SMS based system failed to get sufficient acceptance and coverage within the country (Castro, 2013), and before that the WHO introduced an EpiInfo based system that also fizzled out after a few years.

The continued attention and investment by the NTD department to again introduce an information system despite previous failures, is evidence of a growing realization within the department of the importance of good information and its relevance to the program outcomes.

It also represents an important opportunity to introduce learning from previous attempts and to build learning opportunities into the development and roll-out process.

The following are some lessons learned from the previous attempts to introduce an information system for leprosy.

Lessons learned from previous leprosy information systems in Mozambique

As mentioned above, there are certain factors as identified by Lippeveld, et al. (2000) that often lead to a failure of the Health Information System within such contexts. Within the Mozambique context there have been three previous information systems, namely the current paper based system, an EpiInfo based system, and an SMS based system.

The paper-based information system has never been formally evaluated although some of the aspects noted below were also mentioned by Castro (2013) in his evaluation of a later SMS based leprosy information system in Mozambique. Most of the points below come from the author´s personal experience and observations in support of the leprosy control program between 2004 and 2019.

4.2 Big book – paper-based Leprosy registers

Fragmented database - The paper register-based systems were spread over all the districts, so it was very difficult to have a concise picture of what was happening in the overall picture. This also influenced the flow of data between different administrative levels (Castro, 2013) and highlighted the **need for a single centralized database**.

Difficult access to data – Even if all the books' registers were together in one place, it is a very cumbersome task to count them all up while at the same time dis-aggregating the data according to gender, age and leprosy type. Also, if another more specific data set was needed you had to start the process again. District supervisors only had their small window on the data, and provincial supervisors only had doubtful aggregate data. So, all levels were dis-empowered, and this did not encourage **more in-depth analysis** to identify problems that needed action or correction when overall indicators showed that there was a problem. The lesson here is that **access to data at all levels is a key ingredient to improve data quality and use**.

Doubts about data quality – As the analysis of data in the leprosy registers is a very cumbersome task and requires the presence of the physical book, it is very hard to verify the quality of the data. In some cases, the book is also not filled in well or the data is incomplete. The high staff turnover of supervisors adds to the problem as the primary data source, the patient clinic card, and is frequently not filled in correctly due to a lack of training. The lack of verification has always left provincial and national data analysts very frustrated and skeptical. **Ways should be created to verify the data quality**.

Fixed reporting periods and reporting delays – Provincial and national data analysts gave supervisors a certain cut-off date each trimester by which they have to submit the compiled aggregate data. They complained, however, that most provinces were late in sending the data. From the district supervisors' point of view, after sending in the trimester data report, they were unsure how to handle additional information that came in after the report had already been sent even though it should actually have been included in that time period. This led to data either being added to the next reporting period or just being ignored. In this way reports received on national level were already outdated by the time they were compiled. **Real time data input analysis is needed**.

Cost – Paper registers are fairly cheap to produce and distribute. The costs of meetings however add considerably to the total cost to gather all the registers in one place to verify data or to analyse the data from them. In many of the provinces there was no funding available to have these regular meetings with district supervisors, and therefore provincial supervisors just received the numbers from districts without the possibility to verify them. **The total cost of maintaining a HIS should be taken into consideration**.

Data security – Book registers have a normal life of at least 5 years, but with frequent use the registers can lose their front covers and pages get increasingly dilapidated. Some book registers have been lost to fires or have been damaged by rainwater. **Data needs to be kept securely.**

4.3 WHO – EpiInfo data collection

Around 2007, the WHO attempted to introduce a new country wide information system for leprosy, based on EpiInfo.

Notification forms were distributed to all the districts and district supervisors were trained to fill-in these for each new case of leprosy diagnosed. An automatic carbon copy was kept in the patient file and the original sent to the provincial supervisor.

All provincial supervisors were equipped with a laptop and trained to enter the data onto an EpiInfo data capture sheet on the laptop. A standardized numbering system was also introduced. Provincial supervisors were trained to use the system and also how to extract reports from the system using the EpiInfo data analysis tools. Supervisors then had to create 3-month reports from the data every trimester and send it to Maputo where it was aggregated with data from other provinces. Unfortunately, an evaluation was never done to determine why the EpiInfo based system failed but the author was involved in assisting the provinces with the implementation of the system and the following problems contributed to the ultimate discontinuation of the system:

Data quality issues

The supervisors complained that the notification forms sent from the district supervisors did not always reach their destination, were at times not filled in correctly or were incomplete. As the district supervisor was not close-by, it was difficult to verify the data. There was also no feedback mechanism for the supervisors to confirm if data was received or not. The provincial supervisor did not know the localities indicated by the district supervisors who did not write very clearly, so the provincial supervisors ended up guessing where there was incomplete information. **The need for data verification and quality is again highlighted.**

Data analysis issues

Although the EpiInfo system had very powerful data analysis tools, it was not very user friendly, especially for those not used to electronic data management systems. The national data analysis team also had no way of verifying the data sent to them from the provinces or had difficulty in integrating slightly different versions from different provinces. **Correct versioning and data base design at the start is important.**

Feedback

District supervisors did not receive feedback from the system, and it ended up being a one way sending of information for them. **Feedback** is needed.

Data security

Data was kept on laptops without a backup policy and more than one set of data was lost due to breakdowns or loss of laptops. **Data security and backups are essential.**

4.4 SMS based leprosy information system

Between 2007 and 2012 an SMS based system was developed to try and overcome some of the shortcomings of both the paper-based system and the EpiInfo system.

The SMS based system consisted of a small laptop connected with modems able to receive structured SMS case notifications from district supervisors. The information was stored in a central database and the information made available to the supervisors through SMS and email. There was an attempt to expand the system to the whole country, but it never achieved enough acceptance and the health department did not take full ownership of it.

An evaluation of the system was done by Swiss TPH in 2012 (Castro, 2013) and the following lessons can help guide future information systems in this context:

Integration with other systems

Even though the system used open source tools, it was difficult to **integrate the database into existing health information architectures** of the health department in the country.

Life cycle management

"The formalization of the application governance, development and maintenance, through improving documentation (such as creating an administration manual), plus developing and applying procedures for areas such as issue management, security management and disaster recovery, among others, would increase SMS-Hub maintainability, crucial for further sustainability of the application."(Castro, 2013, p. 5)

Basic policies and procedures for routine management of the system is needed.

Data privacy

As the system used un-encrypted messages and stored patient files in plain text, there was not **sufficient protection of patient data**.

User proficiency and technical support

Using the system was not easy and as there was a high staff turnover, the supervisors required more training. The health department did not have **sufficient technical support and resources** to support the maintenance of the system and the users.

Improved management of leprosy

It can be stated without any doubt that the project improved the management of leprosy in Mozambique, as "accuracy, reliability and availability of leprosy control information" shared between levels of care clearly improved, according to the stakeholders interviewed." (Castro, 2013)

Data quality and improved access can contribute to better leprosy management.

System generated standard reports

It was noted in the evaluation that official reports were easier to generate without previous manual data aggregation which especially made it easier for provincial supervisors to generate shareable reports. It also saved costs and workload in the **transmission of information between district and provincial levels**.

Mobile device management

The project did not purchase any mobile devices for users and they were very comfortable using their own mobile devices for leprosy notifications.

"As a result of the decision to not purchase mobile phones, usual problems in similar projects related to equipment security and accountability of users over assets were not an issue." (Castro, 2013, p. 14)

A **contextualized mobile device management strategy** can contribute to better sustainability.

The above experiences give us valuable contextualized lessons on introducing an information system for the NTD care sector. It is also an introduction to the historical context of the NTD program in Mozambique.

4.5 History and context of the Leprosy and the neglected tropical diseases program within Mozambique

The National Leprosy Control Program is a very old program started in colonial times in

Mozambique. It has been a vertical program under the Infectious Diseases Department and was initially associated with the tuberculosis control program and known as PNCTL (National TB and Leprosy Control Program). After the introduction of Multi Drug Therapy (MDT) and standard fixed regime treatments for Leprosy in the 1980s, treatment coverage was rolled out to all of the country and all of the chronic lifelong patients received a medical cure of the infection for the first time. During this time, the system of patient cards and notification registers was also revived, and some standard indicators introduced by the WHO. A system of provincial and district supervisors were introduced and made responsible for the program implementation and monitoring. During this time the program had support from the WHO and many leprosy related NGOs worldwide were supporting the rollout of the program. Prevalence rates started dropping and in May of 1991 the World Health Assembly adopted a resolution for the elimination of leprosy by 2000, defined as less than one case per 10´000 of the population. The hope was that the transmission of leprosy would be broken, and the disease would slowly disappear.

Mozambique achieved elimination on a country level in 2008 and afterwards a lot of the funding and program focus was diverted to other pressing priorities.

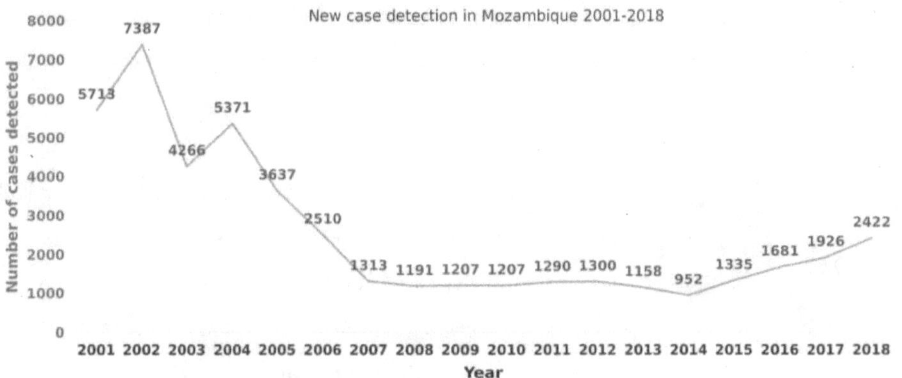

Illustration 9: New case detection in Mozambique 2001-2018 - NTD-Dept report

As can be seen from the National Leprosy Case Detection statistics in the above illustration, before elimination, the country diagnosed more than 4000 new cases annually, the majority of which were in the northern provinces. The case detection rate dropped dramatically up to the elimination point, but then stabilized at around 1200 new cases annually. In the subsequent years, the disability rate started climbing slowly, indicating that leprosy is being diagnosed later in the disease cycle. The percentage of new cases among children also began rising, indicating that the transmission of the disease was still continuing at community level.

From 2010 onward, the profile of Neglected Tropical Diseases was boosted, and the National Leprosy Program was placed under the NTD department. In some provinces the association with tuberculosis was also changed, with leprosy associated more with the Neglected Tropical Diseases Department on district and provincial levels with separate supervisors for NTDs and separate supervisors for Tuberculosis. There has, however, not been a uniform approach to this, and provincial and pistrict health departments have been making their own plans as the prevalence of NTDs and leprosy is also not uniformly distributed throughout the country.

In general, the Leprosy Control Program has lost a lot of focus and quality after elimination was reached. The same was also true for many other countries that have reached the elimination target and have subsequently relaxed their leprosy control activities (Smith et al., 2015).

> *"This decline includes reduced intensity and coverage of case detection activities, community awareness, and training in the diagnosis and treatment of leprosy often associated with the move from vertical leprosy control activities to integrated approaches."*
>
> (Smith et al., 2015, p. 2)

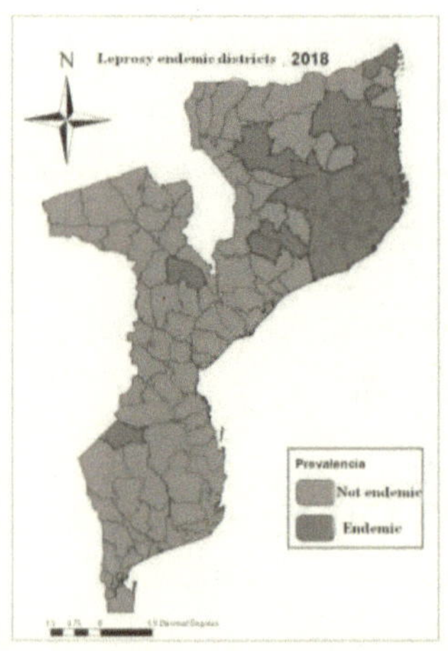

Illustration 10: Districts where leprosy was still endemic by end 2018

From 2012 it became clear that the transmission of leprosy was still continuing and that new case detection rates were beginning to rise, despite weak active case finding initiatives. Since then the case detection has increased annually to over 2400 new cases in 2018. The following illustration demonstrates the distribution of the leprosy burden in Mozambique by 2018. In 2014, the WHO and other partners initiated a plan to stimulate active case finding and improve the quality of the program. As part of this plan, it was suggested to also improve the information system of the Leprosy Control Program and map new cases of leprosy to village level. The development of this new health information system for Leprosy started in 2017 and this study forms part of the efforts to incorporate previous lessons and experiences.

4.6 Implementation process for the DHIS2 based leprosy notification system

This study coincided with the implementation of a HIS implementation project related to NTDs in Mozambique. The objective of the project was to modernize the NTD notification and information system from a paper-based system to a more integrated DHIS2 based system. It also involved the mapping of all secondary data from leprosy and complications of Lymphatic Filariasis (LF) to village level for the past 3-5 years, using the new information system. This project was planned and executed along with the Mozambique Health Department, and insights gained from interviews, meetings, and analysis of the system data was fed back into the implementation process where possible, to contribute to cycles of action learning as the basis for this study and its results.

The project was implemented in three phases, namely the project inception, platform development and testing, and finally the countrywide rollout. Data was gathered during each of these phases and will be presented in subsequent chapters. Here follows a description of the process adopted for each phase of implementation.

4.6.1 Inception

The project started with an inception workshop that was held in August of 2017. A wide range of stakeholders participated during this workshop including representation from all provinces and relevant government departments, including the National Statistical Institute (INE) and National Health Institute (INS). During the workshop the main objectives were determined and a basic plan for implementation was drawn up. A session was also held to inform participants about basic systems thinking as well as a description of the process of Soft Systems Methodology (SSM) that was to be followed during the implementation of the project.

Participants all contributed to the drawing up of a comprehensive **rich picture** of the system from the different points of reference represented during the meeting. **Individual interviews** were also conducted with many of the participants during this meeting, including provincial supervisors and national level data technicians in the NTD department.

The National NTD department took a high level of ownership of the process and actively participated in and facilitated various sessions.

4.6.2 Platform development, Testing and Piloting

In conjunction with relevant stakeholders a framework was drawn up for the new proposed NTD information system specifying the initial requirements.

The following objectives were set for the project implementation:

1. Adequate management and coordination structures are in place for project management and reporting.
2. An Integrated Information System aligned to the National Health System is implemented, and able to produce important management information on cases of leprosy, trachoma and complications of lymphatic filariasis by the end of December 2017.
3. Leprosy, complications of LF and Trachoma Trichiasis are mapped country wide up to the village level where possible, using secondary data, by the end of June 2018.
4. Results are adequately evaluated and the learning shared, leading to the development of a national integrated management plan for the improved management of these cases by the end of June 2018.

One of the initial requirements was compatibility with the current health department HIS which is based on the DHIS2 system. It was felt that some mobile DHIS2 based solution would probably be the most viable, even though the NTD health department team at that stage had a very limited knowledge of DHIS2 systems. The DHIS2 platform had two main infrastructures for mobile data collection, the Tracker Capture and the Events Capture systems. A local company was found that had been the main developers of the DHIS2 system for the Health Department and they agreed to get involved to develop a basic test system to get a feel for how the system was to work. At this stage we discovered that the WHO has also been developing a mobile DHIS2 platform for data collection of CM-NTDs including leprosy. It seemed that the system had much the same objectives as our proposed system and the WHO team was very open to share their work so that we could adapt what they have developed.

The WHO framework was mainly based on the Tracker Capture platform, but they also had some use of Events Capture to import existing data. The Tracker Capture platform is more geared towards continued disease tracking over time, a little like an online patient record system. It has a greater footprint in terms of hardware requirements and bandwidth capacity in comparison to the Events Capture platform. The Events platform is more geared to capturing specific once off data elements as they happen, but still allowed the editing or completion of data already captured, afterwards. It could also be used offline to capture data and when users had the opportunity to go online, the data was synchronized with the main server. It has less demanding bandwidth requirements and the mobile application is able to be installed on most Android phones.

Both the Tracker and Events platforms had a mobile data collection platform available that was actively developed by the DHIS2 community, and it was sufficiently simple and configurable to the local context. The DHIS2 platform also had the ability to map data and create visual reports with GIS coordinates. Partners were sought where the capacity was lacking within the Health Department, for instance, there was nobody that had experience in using GIS systems, and the data was simply not available within the Health Department.

Initially we relied on some older GIS information from third parties that was available for most of the villages in Mozambique. We adapted this data to be integrated into the DHIS2 system. It soon became apparent however that we would have to use more updated and verified information especially if the information is to be accepted officially by the health department. A lot of the historic data and names of villages or administrative areas had already changed, so we had to find a better source of GIS information. The most up to date information in the country was with the National Statistical Institute (INE), who completed a census of the country in 2017 during which they recorded field GPS coordinates. The NTD department made a formal request for a partnership with INE which was approved. It turned out to be a good partnership as we not only received the latest GIS information, but a GIS technician also accompanied our field rollout program and was able to make on the spot corrections to the database or include different levels of localities in accordance with the needs of the supervisors in the provinces and districts.

By this time the DHIS2 development team had also learned how to better integrate the GIS information in the Events user platform so that users can more easily select the village from their

district without having to browse through all of the available localities.
After the initial platform was developed it was decided to run pilots in a less endemic province (Gaza) and a more endemic province (Cabo Delgado). This was done in November of 2017. During the pilot studies, further interviews were also done with district supervisors.
The following lessons were learned during the two pilot studies:

General - Planning and coordination

It was noted that there was very little secondary Trichiasis data available and it was felt that this component should be taken out of the objectives. The initial proposed rollout strategy of training trainers and then having a decentralized rollout was deemed impractical. Many adaptations have had to be made on the spot, for instance, GIS verification and corrections to the platform, or hardware errors, that a lone provincial supervisor would not be able to handle on his own. As the rollout strategy would require more technical assistance from a centralized team, the timeline and budget for the project needed to be adapted.

Mobile platform and equipment

After the pilot studies, it was felt that the phones used did not respond well to the needs of the project. A bigger screen would give easier access to the forms, and better battery life would help. It was also felt that the terms of reference for the equipment needs review to minimize risks like changes in staff, breakages etc.
It was known that the TB program was also planning to buy tablets for their mobile data collection using Tracker. The team proposed to seek partnerships with this program so as not to duplicate resources. Hardware and data security were very weak and needed to be improved. A process was started to investigate Mobile Device Management (MDM) options and to develop better policies for this.

Application development and GIS integration.

Many small adaptations were made to the Events platform user interface after getting feedback from the users in the meeting after the pilot was completed.
The importance of good GIS data was highlighted, and it was proposed to create a working relationship with INE to try and integrate updated data after the 2017 census. The structure of the

data of INE was, however, different from the organizational structure used in SISMA (DHIS2 MOH server). In particular, for SISMA, information may be needed as to which villages and areas are allocated to each Health post. This information was not readily available in the MOH and may need to be defined in the future.

There was also some difficulty in integrating the case-based data in the main aggregate SISMA server. Personnel from the department running the main SISMA (DHIS2) server of the Health Department was only occasionally involved and did not effectively have input into the design and learning during the pilot projects and roll-out of the system. Full integration was not achieved by the end of the project.

Data quality, indicators and user feedback

Some progress was made in defining the LF data flow structure and the data gathering tools.

It was noted that there was a need to try to verify data quality during the process where possible.

Indicators needed to be defined in the DHIS2 platform as well as reports for various levels of users.

Work was started on the Dashboard mobile platform for user feedback.

It was noted that in most Districts (except in Cabo Delgado) the leprosy and TB programs were run by one supervisor and the NTD program by another. Some pros and cons of this were discussed but no consensus reached.

User maintenance and sustainability

It was noted that the MOH was developing longer-term plans to supply internet facilities to the provincial and district services and possibly up to health post level. In the meantime, a solution was needed to supply internet to district users on a regular basis within the limits of the project. It was important to define the limits of this commitment so that sustainability in the long-term is not compromised. The need was also noted to maintain a central register of user numbers and equipment.

Evaluation, Lessons learned and Training development.

The team felt that learning gained during the pilot phase needed to be captured and material prepared for the rollout to other provinces so that lessons could be incorporated. It was suggested that Video tutorials could be used as a training tool.

The above lessons were discussed during a follow-up planning meeting with partners in February of 2018. During this opportunity input was also gained in reflecting on the previously made **rich pictures** and the group contributed to the development of **root definitions** to describe the objective of the system.

4.6.3 Field rollout, training and follow-up

Various changes to the software and mobile infrastructure were introduced after feedback from the pilot studies. A next group of provinces were then selected, and the system introduced in Inhambane, Manica, Sofala, Nampula and Zambezia. With each consecutive province, the data entry took less time and errors were identified and rectified.

During a field rollout a meeting area was selected that had good cell phone reception, as it was needed for the participants to link to the internet in order to update the meta-data initially. A username and password were created for each user beforehand, and users was asked to buy a SIM card prior to the meeting. The workshop was arranged for 3-4 days, depending on the number of districts in the province, and the amount of secondary data that had to be introduced.

The rollout workshop program followed roughly the following structure:

Day 1

1. Presentation of the objectives of the workshop.
2. Presentations on the leprosy and the NTD situation from at least the most endemic districts and the province. This provided a good overview of the level and quality of data available in the province, and some other issues that may be relevant, such as the level of training of the district supervisors or specific program issues that may have an influence on the later use of the system and data.
3. Situation of leprosy and other NTDs at a national level. Participants are made aware of the bigger context of NTDs in the country.
4. An explanation of the objectives and the user policy of the tablet being given. The rules of use of the equipment being provided is explained and users are made aware of some of the risks and limitations.
5. Distribution of the tablets to the districts. - Users have to sign the TOR for the use of the tablets.

6. An explanation of the use of the tablet. - It is explained how to switch on, charge the tablets, and take care of the equipment. Users are linked to the internet. The cell phone company provided 5 Gigabytes of data to users with new SIM cards. Where needed, we gave some users phone credit to convert to data packages.
7. Introduction to the installation and use of the DHIS2 platform. A locally modified version of the DHIS2 Events platform was previously loaded onto the tablets. An f-droid repository was also activated, as we did not want users to install the version available on the internet. This is shown to the users in case the system gets uninstalled for some reason in the future. We also encouraged users to install the platform on their own Android phone as a backup.
8. Demonstration on the use of the DHIS2 platform.
   A tablet was linked with Airdroid or Vysor to a PC and the screen shared and projected for all to follow the process better. Users was stepped through the process of how to enter data into the system.
9. Practice in the use of the platform with a "demo" account.
   A "demo" user account was shared with users which they could use to practice introducing data into the system. Some cases were entered by all users using all the same village and the results then projected to demonstrate errors and how to correct them.

Day 2

1. Data management and data quality in the leprosy and NTD sector.
   Users were reminded of the process of data flow in the system and encouraged to compare secondary sources with the primary sources to assure data is complete and correct. Both the Leprosy and Lymphatic Filariasis (LF) data sources were reviewed.
2. Introduction to GIS data used in the DHIS2 system.
   The division of districts into localities and villages is very complex, and some limits had to be set on which location levels could be included in the platform to keep it as complete yet manageable possible. It was also explained that the names that people called villages may not be the official name in the state register.
3. Sharing of the usernames and passwords of district supervisors.
   Users received their own login and passwords which were then introduced. Where needed errors were corrected on the spot in the main system to get user accounts active.

4. Start the input of secondary data by users in the DHIS2 platform.

   As there was districts with lots of data and districts with few data, teams were made by grouping high and low endemic districts. The process flowed much quicker by having one person read the data from the register and the other imputing it in the DHIS2 platform. After some time, they could swap roles. We started with the most recent data and worked our way backwards to as far back as data was available or that time allowed.

Day3 and 4

1. Continue to introduce secondary data.

   Participants continued to introduce data. From time to time the process was interrupted to get a general feel where the group was in the process and to highlight specific errors to avoid or correct. Some goals were also set for the days' work when we saw that participants got very distracted or unfocused.
2. Introduction to the lymphatic filariasis (LF) data platform.

   By this time users were very familiar with the platform and it was easy to introduce them to the LF data capture side of the platform. This followed the same conventions as the Leprosy side and are much shorter and simpler that the leprosy side, so users quickly got the hang of it. In most cases the participants did not have LF data available to introduce but was encouraged to do so when they had access to this data back in their districts.
3. Feedback and reports from the DHIS2 system.

   By this time all districts have managed to enter at least 1 to 2 years' worth of data in the system. The DHIS2 system also had time to synchronize data to the reporting side of the system to visualize the data.

   Dashboards were created in the DHIS2 platform for each district user separately and a standard set of predefined reports were loaded. These reports were mostly bar-charts of new cases diagnosed per year or quarter, number of men and women diagnosed, number of new cases with deformity, etc. We also included a map of each district showing the location of notified cases and a list of all cases registered.

   Users were then introduced to the DHIS2 Interactive Dashboard application from HISP Tanzania that was found to better visually represent the DHIS2 data. Users used the same login and password to get access to their DHIS2 platform using this system. Reports from one of the districts were again projected to show users how the system works and demonstrate the significance of the reports. Users are then asked to verify the reports by comparing them to the number of cases that were notified to date.

4. Verification of the data entered so far.
   This was done especially in conjunction with the provincial supervisor who had to learn how to access reports and detailed lists on the Web platform in order to verify the data for completeness and quality, from the district supervisors.
   The book registers of each district were compared line by line with the electronic data and where found errors were corrected.
5. Introduction to other systems installed on the tablets: SkinApp, Fdroid and Miradore.
   Some other applications were also installed on the tablets. They included SkinApp, which is a medical application helping clinicians make a better differential diagnosis for leprosy and other skin diseases by using a search function for typical symptoms and pictures of typical cases.
   Fdroid was also installed as a repository for our version of the DHIS2 Events Capture platform and to share other resources in the future with users, such as a user manual which was not yet available.
   A mobile device management (MDM) application Miradore was also activated on all tablets and users informed about the need for this and ways we could use it if tablets were stolen or lost, etc.

This concludes a description of the process that were followed to install a new information system for leprosy and other neglected tropical diseases in Mozambique. The process took nearly 18 months to complete and many lessons were subsequently fed back into the development and rollout processes. The following chapters will detail some of the specific findings and learning that came out of the Soft Systems Methodology (SSM) used during the process.

4.7 Soft System Methodology – actual situation – rich pictures

The objective of the rich pictures was to get an overview of all the players involved in the system and the ways that they relate to each other. It can also highlight certain choke points or conflicts areas, and already serves as an intervention to stimulate debate on these issues.

During a series of interviews with various stakeholders, individually and also in a group setting during meetings, the participants made a pictorial representation of their system, and the stakeholders and procedures within those systems. The most comprehensive one was during the inception workshop involving most of the provincial leprosy supervisors as well as national NTD program staff and incorporated the perspectives of various levels in the leprosy care system from the village level up to the National level. During this meeting the participants were asked to draw the NTD care system on a big sheet of paper and it was subsequently discussed, and additions made to add more detail or highlight specific issues.

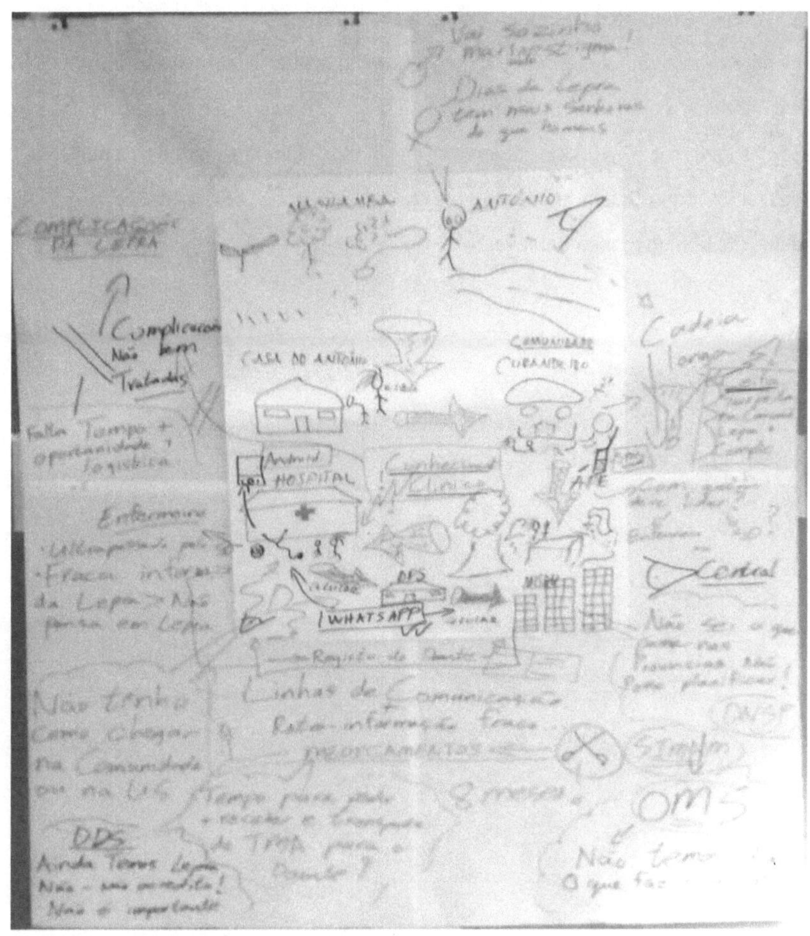

Illustration 11: Original Rich picture of the leprosy care system

The rich picture that was made during the inception workshop tells the story of a fictional man Antonio. He is typically a subsistence farmer that is unaware that he has leprosy. His wife notices that he has some skin patches. Their first port of call is the traditional healer, who does not recognize leprosy but asks them money for treatment that does not work. Some time goes by, but the situation gets worse. Fortunately, there is a leprosy community volunteer that is contacted at some stage, andhe examines Antonio and suspects that it is leprosy. He directs Antonio to the nearest health post where a nurse examines him. She unfortunately has not been trained in leprosy or does not have a lot of clinical experience in leprosy and fails initially to make the diagnosis. After some more wasted time and insistence from the community volunteer the leprosy district supervisor is informed and after some time comes to that area and finally manages to diagnose leprosy and start treatment. Often the community volunteer would even bypass the health post nurse completely and go directly to the district supervisor. The district supervisor then records the information as a new case in the patient register and from time to times sends aggregate data to the provincial level that eventually sends the information up to national level.

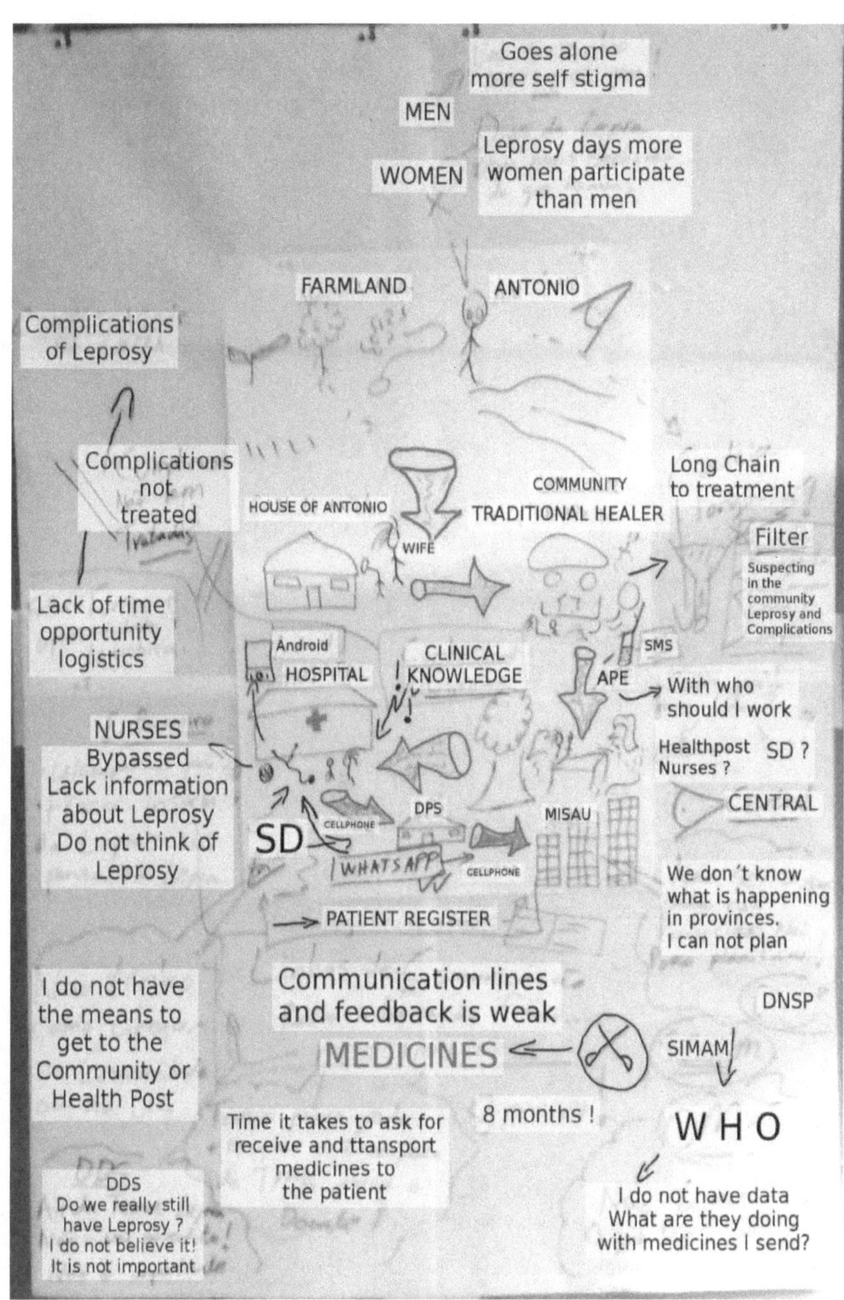

Illustration 12: Translated Rich picture of the leprosy care system

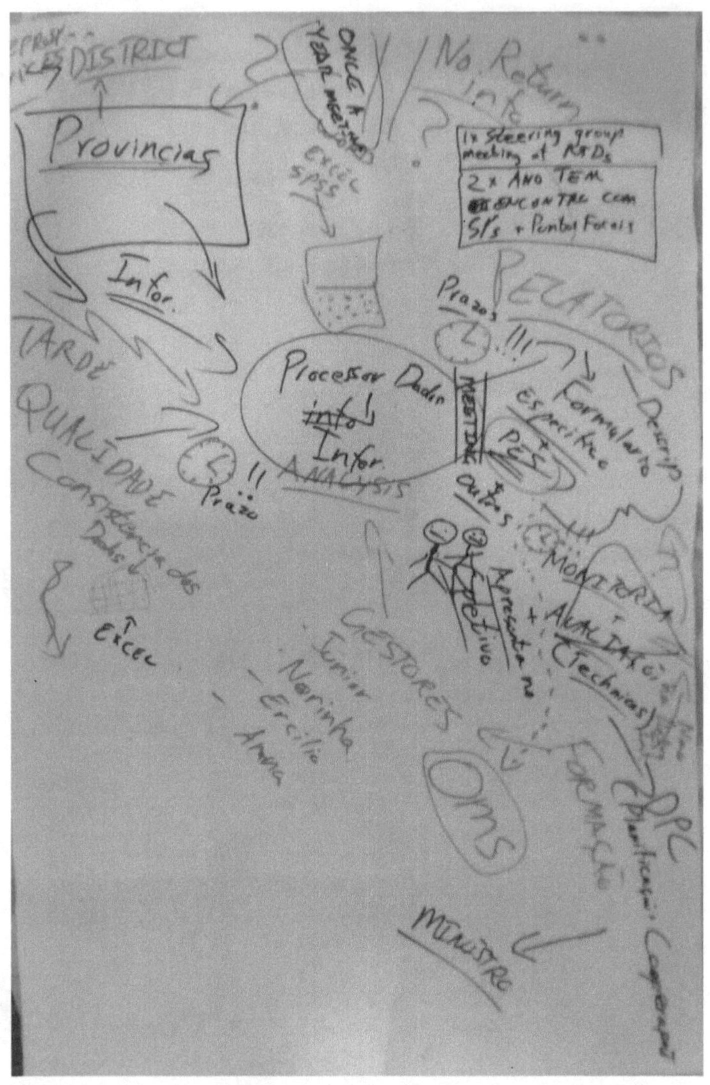

Illustration 13: Original Rich picture of national leprosy data analysis team

A similar analysis and rich picture was made during a separate meeting with the national leprosy data processing team. On national level there was a very different story unfolding and a whole new set of issues that come into play. At this level the main issue was having reliable and timely information to make decisions and supply the resources needed for the program, particularly medicines. Reports also needed to go to various state departments and the WHO, who also questioned the validity of the information etc.During individual interviews with supervisors, they were also asked to draw a picture of how they saw their work-system. The objective was to verify the rich picture from the bigger group and also to see if there are may be other important issues from their perspectives.

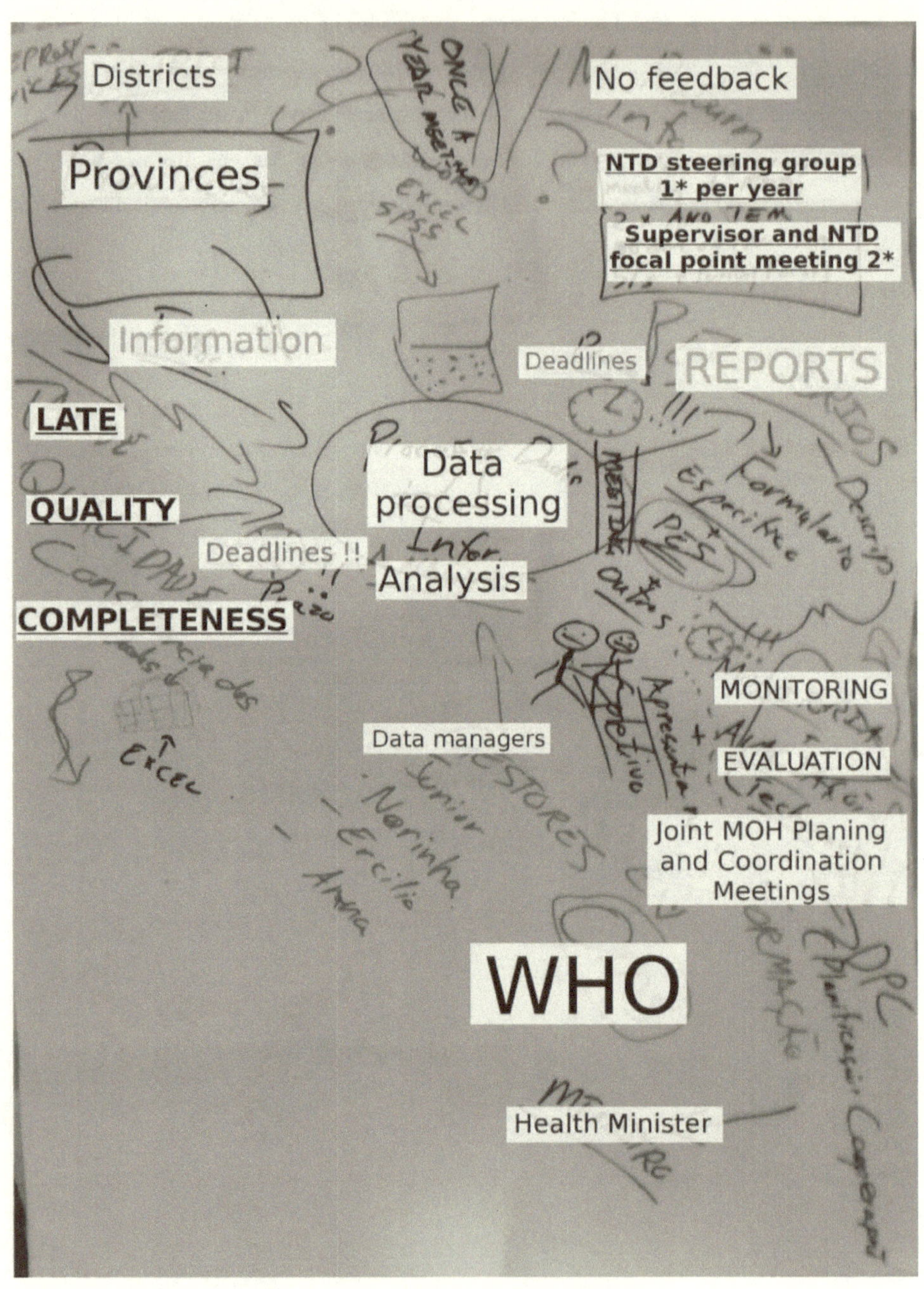

Illustration 14: Translated rich picture of national data collection team

The pictures from the district and provincial supervisors did not add much new information and seemed to confirm our understanding from the bigger rich picture.
The rich picture from the national level data analysts was a bit more interesting and showed a lot of the dynamic on the national level with the pressures and interactions that exist there. The picture was full of clocks symbolizing the pressure to deliver information within deadlines. It also highlighted the apparent lack of feedback, to the provincial and district levels, of the results of the data analysis, and the apparent disconnect between the clinical and epidemiological situation in the districts and the how the data was visualized on national level. It did not seem that epidemiological trends or red flags could easily inform practice and priorities on the district clinical level.
In general, though, the initial rich picture created during the bigger group meeting seemed to be a good representation of the NTD care system to date.

4.8 Soft System Methodology – actual situation – stakeholder interviews

Interviews were arranged with various stakeholders during the rollout process, utilizing various opportunities during meetings or field visits. Provincial and district supervisors were chosen that had some experience in the program, as there is a high turnover, especially of district supervisors, the perspectives were sought of those that had a better understanding of the running of the system. The provincial supervisor was asked to select the district supervisors most suited in terms of experience. Making a random selection of supervisors would not add much value at this point as it was more important to get appropriate data and get a general perspective of how the system worked for the SSM process. Interviews were held with stakeholders from the north, center and south of the country representing a higher and lower endemic perspective. Four district supervisors were interviewed as well as three provincial supervisors.
A suitable space was arranged for having a good conversation, and after permission was obtained, the interview was recorded in audio format.
The same interview framework was used during all interviews, starting by asking participants to describe the typical activities they do each day, then branching to other areas like the resources they used, and the objectives, final outcomes, and successes that they want to see in their work. The participants were also asked, at the end of the interview, to draw a picture of how their system

worked, on a large piece of paper with some markers provided.

After the interviews, the aspects expressed by the participants were summarized in the interview framework structure. The interview results from all the interviews were then listed in a consolidated interview framework list using the same structure. Common themes were then identified in the consolidated framework lists and grouped. The objective was not to do a statistical analysis, but to understand the system from the perspective of the interviewed supervisors. A separate breakdown was done for district and provincial supervisors.

Consolidated interview results for district supervisors

District Supervisors - Resources / Input (What resources / inputs do I need to do my job?)			
	Theme	Count	%
1	Communication means / channels	8	26%
2	Transport / logistical support	7	23%
3	Community partners (to help with my work)	4	13%
4	Registers / cards / forms	3	10%
5	Other (eg PPDs and lab diagnostic tools)	3	10%
6	Medicines to treat patients (MDT)	2	6%
7	Incentives / funds	2	6%
8	Training (funds and training materials for nurses)	2	6%
	TOTAL	31	

District Supervisors – Activities (What do I do every day ?)			
	Theme	Count	%
1	Supervision / Technical support (Monitoring and Evaluation...)	11	19%

2	Active case finding / clinical work (eg. examining patients)	10	17%
3	Training, Health Education and awareness	10	17%
4	Coordination with partners / Meetings	8	14%
5	Other / unrelated (eg. get feedback from Volunteers)	8	14%
6	Data gathering and analysis (eg. Fill in patient cards and register and analyse data)	7	12%
7	Planning / Control resources (eg. ask for transport and medicines)	3	5%
8	TB Lab smears	2	3%
	TOTAL	59	

District Supervisors – Background/Conflict/Vision (What helps or hinders your work ?)		
	Recurrent Themes	Count
1	Lack of funds / resources in Leprosy / personnel / transport (hinders my work)	8
2	Reports / indicators and feedback help orientate my work (helps my work)	8
3	Partnerships are important for success (helps my work)	7
4	Weak spot at healthpost/peripheral level in diagnosis / followup. (lack of capacity there hinders my work)	4
5	I do not have time to do fieldwork (hinders my work)	3

District Supervisors - Objectives (Why - Transformation and **Weltanschhaung**?) (Why do I do what I do ?)		
	Recurrent Themes	Count
1	Disease related - Attain objectives / indicators "Come to an end of these illnesses" "Transform the problem that brought people to hospital"	8
2	Shared ownership / partnerships / Coordination "if the team works well then my work is easier" "or we do not involve them, they will not follow our advice and services and the problem will remain"	4
3	Personal satisfaction "Suspect cases and are able to diagnose new cases gives me satisfaction"	3
4	Raise awareness / educate	3

Table 5: Consolidated interview results for district supervisors

Consolidated interview results for provincial supervisors

Provincial Supervisors - Resources / Input

(What resources / inputs do I need to do my job?)

	Theme	Count	%
1	Communication means / channels	8	44%
2	Transport (eg. motorbike or fuel to get places)	4	22%
3	Registers / cards / forms	4	22%
4	Medicines for patients (MDT)	1	6%
5	Incentives for Community volunteers	1	6%

Provincial Supervisors – Activities (What do I do every day ?)

	Theme	Count	%
1	Supervision / Technical support (Monitoring and Evaluation...)	10	29%
2	Coordination with partners / Meetings (with other partners or district supervisors)	9	26%
3	Data gathering and analysis (eg. get data from supervisors, compile and send etc.)	5	15%
4	Active case finding / clinical work (eg. contact tracing)	4	12%
5	Training (eg. train nurses or supervisors)	4	12%
6	Control resources (eg. control MDT stock level)	1	3%
7	Planning (in general)	1	3%

Provincial Supervisors – Background/Conflict/Vision
(What helps or hinders your work ?)

	Recurrent Themes	Count
1	Lack of funds / resources in Leprosy (hinders my work)	6
2	Training needs not adequately addressed “Even the Provincial Supervisor has a lack of information on Leprosy - the SDs even more” (hinders our work)	6
3	Data gathering for reports / indicators difficult / frustrating “What pressures me most is to control the data that I receive from the districts” “The problem is with the data gathering at the primary data source”	6
4	TB program requires more attention and time (hinders leprosy work)	3

Provincial Supervisors - Objectives (Why - Transformation and **Weltanschhaung**?) - (Why do I do what I do ?)		
	Recurrent Themes	Count
1	Improve outcomes / reach goals	7
2	Data quality and analysis (eg. to identify problems that needs addressing)	2

Table 6: Consolidated interview results for provincial supervisors

4.9 Complimentary data – Document analysis

The purpose of the document analysis is firstly to help verify the observations made during the situation analysis and rich picture creation and to identify other aspects of the NTD care system that may not have been identified.

Secondly, the documents may also help to identify any aspects or lack of aspects related to knowledge management in the NTD care system. For this, the performance measurement framework adapted by Faisst and Resatsch (2004) was used as a way to group issues that indicate the effectiveness of knowledge management during the time of the project roll-out. This could also indicate specific issues that are needed to improve knowledge management in the future.

This knowledge management framework as also set out in section 3.4 consists of 4 groups (Classes)

Knowledge base indicators (Class I)

System quality, Knowledge quality (Documents), Knowledge specific service.

This encompasses the systems and infrastructure to capture data and knowledge, to organise and store it.

Cost indicators (Class II)

Costs of interventions, Interceding processes.

Encompasses the costs of running the Knowledge management system. What effort needed to keep it going?

Intermediation and transfer indicators (Class III)

System usage, User satisfaction, Knowledge transfer within the organization.

Is the right knowledge getting to the right places / users ?

Effect indicators on business results (Class IV)

Business results (Health service outcomes)

Is the knowledge changing anything for the better ?

The following types of documentation were available for analysis:

4.9.1 Reports from the pilot studies and rollouts in various provinces

Reports was received from 5 of the 7 provinces where the notification rollout had taken place to date. From these reports, issues related to knowledge management in the NTD care system was identified that existed before the rollout as well as issues that came up during the rollout process. These were then grouped in the performance measurement framework as adapted by Faisst and Resatsch (2004) . Issues mentioned more frequently were listed first:

Knowledge base indicators (Class I) *(Systems and infrastructure)*

- Data and reports sent late to the central NTD department. (4x)
- No automatic numbering of new cases. (2x)
- Medication reports aggregated with other information making it difficult to get a clear picture.
- Districts do not report when medicines run out.
- Some confusion about finding localities in the notification system.
- Trimester meetings in districts for data collection and verification are not regular or are not happening in many provinces.
- Documents and clinic cards are not organized / filed well.
- Poor notification of LF complications even in endemic districts.
- Instruments for collecting other NTD data not in use.

Cost indicators (Class II) *(What effort is needed to keep it going?)*

None

Intermediation and transfer indicators (Class III) (*Is the right knowledge getting to the right places / users ?*)

- Lack of knowledge on leprosy indicators (e.g. Coorts) (4x)
- No feedback sent to provinces from central NTD dept. (4x)
- No feedback sent to the districts from provinces. (2x)
- Provincial supervisors were not proficient in technical areas of the system. (2x)
- Lack of coordination between leprosy and NTD focal points. (2x)
- Lack of in-service training. (2x)
- District supervisors are not proficient with the Excel database.
- No knowledge of endemic hotspots is neighbouring districts, provinces or countries.
- Poor follow-up and technical support to districts.
- Feedback was not given to clinics / districts after hydrocele surgery.

Effect indicators on business results (Class IV) (*Is the knowledge changing anything for the better ?*)

- Poor contact tracing.
- Leprosy drugs expire in low endemic districts.
- Difficulty in diagnosing leprosy early.
- Lack of clinical information on leprosy.
- Lack of material for hydrocele surgery.
- Lack of leprosy medications.
- Poor integration of leprosy with other NTDs.
- Poor involvement of other stakeholders in leprosy detection.

4.9.2 Planning and feedback reports from the information system implementation

This was a consolidated report, produced in February 2018, of issues identified during the rollout process that led to later changes to the system and the implementation process. The report was structured in the following way:

- General – Planning and coordination
- Devises and equipment
- App development and GIS integration
- Data quality, indicators, and user feedback
- User maintenance and sustainability
- Evaluation, lessons learned, and training development
- Proposed timeline until the project ended

The issues identified in the report were again arranged in the performance measurement framework as adapted by Faisst and Resatsch (2004):

Knowledge base indicators (Class I) *(Systems and infrastructure)*

- The importance of functional partnerships with INE (National statistical institute) is identified as a critical aspect to verify and update the GIS database of the health ministry as they are the principal source of GIS data in the country.
- The need to correctly structure and standardize the GIS data for the Health Department is identified as this data is structured differently according to different functional applications in other departments. This decision needs to be taken at the correct level.
- The need for integration into the existing MOH information system is recognized.
- Some partners feel information on hydrocele is not needed as most hydroceles will be resolved in 2 years' time.
- The need for data verification is emphasized.
- Indicators and reports for various levels in the care system are needed and the technical team will start to develop these.

Cost indicators (Class II) *(What effort is needed to keep it going?)*

- The terms of reference for the equipment needs review to minimize risks, like changes in staff, breakages, etc. A new term of reference for staff is needed.
- It is suggested to seek partnerships with the TB program to not duplicate resources like equipment where possible.
- The need for Mobile devise management is identified as well as the development of

appropriate policies and procedures.

- In most provinces the leprosy and TB programs are run by one supervisor and the NTD program by another. This might lead to some duplication of roles and more complicated coordination.
- Sustainability needs to be strongly considered and commitments limited for supplying internet connectivity to users.

Intermediation and transfer indicators (Class III) *(Is the right knowledge getting to the right places / users ?)*

- The Android phones used during the pilots did not respond well to the needs of the project. A little bigger screen would be useful and better battery life would help.
- A central shared repository for Android applications and manuals is needed to standardize installation and use. An F-Droid repository was created.
- Maintaining internet connectivity for users is still a challenge.
- A user register with cell phone numbers and equipment is needed.
- Learning on the implementation process needs to be captured.

Effect indicators on business results (Class IV) *(Is the knowledge changing anything for the better ?)*

None

4.10 Complimentary data – Expert interviews

An opportunity presented itself to learn from other African countries implementing the DHIS2 system during a DHIS2 mobile devise workshop in Zimbabwe during 2018.

The countries of Ghana and Zimbabwe have both implemented successful mobile data gathering DHIS2 systems over the past 3 or more years in the malaria and tuberculosis programs. They have also moved to Android based individual patient data gathering over the past 2 years using the DHIS2 Tracker system, which is similar to the system that was being implemented in Mozambique. An interview was set up with both the Ghana and Zimbabwe project managers to learn from their experiences during this process.

The WHO – MAPS toolkit (mHealth Assessment and Planning for Scale) was used as a basic framework for the interview which was recorded in English.

The following learning points were gathered from these interviews:

4.10.1 Specific learning points from Zimbabwe:

- Training can promote the use of data by users in order to influence decisions.
- Strategic thinking / planning for program goals and outcomes and then the information system is to support that progress. "I think it is starts from strategic thinking, where you say there is a strategic plan in place that has your goals and milestones that you have to get to" (1:03).
- Having tools that are easy to use promotes data use and better decisions.
- A wide participation in seeing the information with the help of tools like dashboards.
- Information, for instance in dashboards, should be easily accessible.
- A scorecard system that can quickly flag something visually when action is needed would help promote data use and decision making. "The whole idea is to stimulate discussion around the information and data that has been sent." (2:12)
- Integrated Disease Surveillance and Response guidelines from the WHO have been used to train personnel in each health facility. "In every health facility there is a person that has been trained on that." (3:54) This helps to give staff thresholds for interpreting the data and taking action. There are also guidelines in which people are trained as to what action to take, for instance, when a new case of malaria is diagnosed, etc.
- Feedback loops at the lower facility level would be useful (even though not yet possible in Zimbabwe).
- Reports based on aggregated data from the system helps change behavior: "But once you study it in a report format the district can easily and quickly see, and if you do these reports people can start to make decisions." (5:58) Data needs to be used...
- Data from the system needs to be used in reports and feedback back to the senders: "...they start to realize that the information that they are sending is being used. And that then makes them compliant to do a better job and they improve their processes." (6:20)
- Various ways can be used to motivate lower level users to take ownership or to comply with the system, namely, financial incentives, continued training, understanding the impact of

their work and the results of the system (self motivation), and proper job descriptions guided by program policies. "They understand the benefit that this one brings as compared to where they were, so I think it is not a one answer but if your capacity build someone enough they understand the objective the endgame and everything. And they think why not let me be part of it." (13:17)

- Users should also be involved in the design of the system from the start. "So it is also the involvement in the design of that system because they are the final users. You do not want to come and dump something just saying this is what you are going to do..." (14:40)
- Governance decisions and policies comes from the higher (central) level and are shared with other level users. "There is no parallel (structure) or anyone implementing some kind of (parallel thing), everything is within an integrated structure." (17:15)
- For routine internet costs the central level sometimes provides some resources, but a lot depends on peoples' intrinsic motivation to take initiatives themselves for a connection.
- For equipment replacement that gets lost there are policies and procedures in place. A committee reviews the circumstances of the loss and makes a verdict.
- Tablets are insured and can be replaced under certain conditions by the insurer.
- A centralized training is usually done first, which is then followed up by a decentralized training of trainers model and then supported by the M&E processes.
- Documentation and detailed manuals should also be available to support training.

4.10.2 Learning points from Ghana

- Alignment of data sets for different stakeholders is important (e.g. donors). It makes integration easier.
- In-house capacity to evaluate their own needs – as their situation and data needs changed, they did their own evaluations and made recommendations to their health department. "We were not open for someone dumping a system on us." (6:55)
- DHIS2 system led to improvements in speed and efficiency of data collection.
- Users are being challenged to base decisions on data. There is a system of regular reviews of performance based on the data from the DHIS2 system. This is done on the different levels of the service hierarchy from the facility level up. Facilities or districts are compared, and this

adds to pressure "... usually at the facility level they think that the data is not theirs, they are only pushing it, but we are gradually getting that to them ..." (10:30) (data ownership and responsibility)

- Feedback is sent down the line based on the DHIS2 and the performance review. "... the district feedback to the various facilities is also very important ..." (11:25)
- It is felt that at the lower (facility) level data ownership and use is improved by helping users visualize and engage with patient level data. "... you are seeing your client level data - he is defaulting ..." (11:10) (Having access to data, visualizing it effectively and getting feedback on specific warning signs and knowing what to do ...)
- There are some predefined operating procedures "... we have a standard operating procedure ..." (12:00) - it needs follow-up ...
- Staff is allocated at various levels in the HIS. The core person to champion and promote the use of the system is however on middle level management: "The core function falls on the district director of the health services" (13:30) who promotes the use of the system, and is alsolinked to supervision and monitoring systems.
- There seems to be an elaborate framework of aligned policies and guidelines supporting the DHIS2 setup: We have an enterprise architecture, (how eHealth should be implemented in Ghana). We have eHealth strategy. We have the HIS policy guidelines. We have the Ghana Health services standard approach and procedure guidelines and Extension and M&E frameworks and others that details what we need to be doing ... - "All of these are in line ..." (14:20)
- Responsibility for the cost for routine access to the DHIS2 server (internet costs) are decentralized and facilities and districts have to plan and budget for this cost. "We have for sustainability sake decentralized the cost of things to the districts." (16:48)
- There seem to be policies in place for equipment use and responsibility. Equipment initially supplied by the central program, but facilities are then responsible for maintenance and replacement of equipment.
- Training is more decentralized - on the job training rather than a centralized form of training. "We decentralize the training as much as possible." (23:25)
- As part of the M&E there are yearly audits of the IT system on various levels.

- Equipment turnover is a challenge and happens every 2-3 years. There are guidelines made for facilities on the equipment and users / managers are taken through the guidelines at the start.
- Community health nurses (paid health-care personnel) are registered on the system, but not community volunteers. This is already a fairly detailed level of service point registration (to lower levels in the hierarchy) on the system.
- Ghana has GIS integration in their system up to the facility level but not to the village level. Villages are assigned to specific facilities which helps to dis-aggregate the data at the facility level if needed.
- People can be encouraged to interact with the data at lower levels in the hierarchy by a system of oversight using the data received to evaluate performance. M&E performance and appraisals need to be used to stimulate people to use the data. "When a subordinate realizes that you are looking at the data they sit up and they start working on that data very well" (35:33)
- Planning and budgeting should happen at the facility level and be based on data from the system, and then be put together at higher levels. "One other thing we are doing in Ghana is that your service data and your budget and your plans should have a co-relation." (36:25) The service data is linked to the Ghana health services objectives, so look at your burden of diseases, and plan where you are allocating your resources accordingly.

4.11 Complimentary data – Technology survey

During the start of the NTD mapping project the NTD department did a small survey to roughly determine the level of connectivity and technology use of the district supervisors in the country. The survey consisted of 9 questions in an excel format that were sent to the Provincial supervisors who was asked to fill it in after consulting with district supervisors.

The results of the survey are summarized in the table below :

ITEM	QUESTIONARIO	NIASSA	CABO DELGADO	NAMPULA	ZAMBEZIA	MANICA	SOFALA	INHAMBANE	GAZA	MAPUTO PROVINCIA	MAPUTO CIDADE
1	How many districts in your Province ?	16	17	23	22	12	13	14	14	8	7
2	How many of the district supervisors have a "SmartPhone"	11	13	19	20	0	13	11	9	7	4
3	How many of the district supervisors use WhatsApp?	10	11	19	20	3	13	11	9	7	3
4	How many district supervisors have an email address?	5	5	19	18	12	11	11	5	6	2
5	Which ceelphone networks do the supervisors use ? Movitel: Mcel : Vodacom:	1 13 2	4 6 7	0 0 23	3 10 9	12 0 0	4 3 6	9 6 10	4 14 6	0 1 7	2 0 5
6	Except for WhatApp, what other social networks do supervisors use?	Facebook	Facebook	Facebook	Facebook	Nenhum	Nenhum	Fecebook,Skype	Nenhum	6	Facebook
7	Acording to your estimate, what % of community volunteers have a cellphone able to send an SMS ?	60%	100%	50%	60%	0%	30%	100%	90%	80%	20%
8	Acording to your estimate, what % of nurses at health-posts have a cellphone able to send an SMS ?	100%	100%	90%	100%	100%	99%	100%	100%	100%	100%
9	Acording to your estimate, what % of nurses at health-posts have a "SmartPhone": ?	60%	40%	20%	90%	0%	99%	100%	80%	60%	65%

Table 7: Results from technology survey Mozambique provinces 2018

4.12 Complimentary data – Health information system data.

As the new HIS started to be used more frequently by the provinces and the health ministry in Maputo was receiving more data on a regular basis, they started various processes to verify the data received. One of the comparisons that the health ministry made, was to look at the data they had available before the new system was introduced and compared it to the data for the same periods and places reported by the DHIS2 system. This was possible as retrospective data for the last 3-5 years was entered for all the provinces where the system was implemented. Previous data was captured in an aggregated form in an Excel data sheets and this was then compared to the aggregated numbers from the DHIS2 system. The results were summarized in the following graphs produced by the health ministry during the project closure meeting.

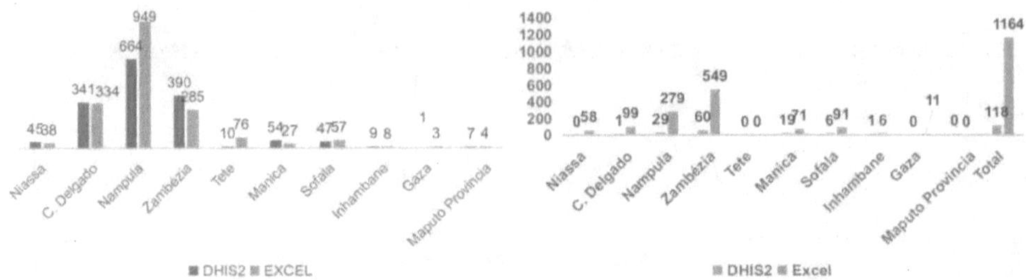

Illustration 15: Discrepancies between Excel and DHIS2 leprosy new case detection numbers for January to August 2018

Illustration 16: Discrepancies between number of lymphedema reported in Excel and DHIS2 for January to August 2018

The health ministry along with some of their partners have also started to experiment with the DHIS2 reporting and mapping capabilities to try and learn from some of the information presented in the maps as illustrated by the following maps produced by them.

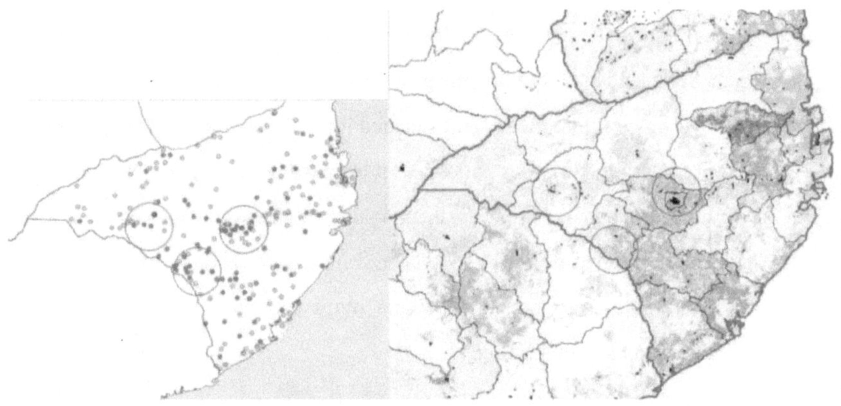

Illustration 17: Distribution of leprosy cases in relation to the population in the Nampula province

5 Analysis

The analysis section is structured in the following way:

5.1 The current state of the HIS and Knowledge Management in the NTD sector in Mozambique.

(In this section the data from the following sections are analyzed and discussed.)

5.1.1 Soft Systems Methodology process – analysis of rich pictures.

5.1.2 Soft Systems Methodology process – analysis of stakeholder interviews.

5.1.3 Document analysis results

5.1.4 Analysis of the technology survey

5.2 What should the aims of the HIS be in the NTD care context in Mozambique based on the specific objectives of the NTD care system.

5.2.1 Soft Systems Methodology process – Input – Output diagrams

5.2.2 Soft Systems Methodology process – CATWOE analysis and root definitions

5.2.3 Soft Systems Methodology process – Conceptual models

5.3 What could a better model for Knowledge Management look like in the real world NTD context in Mozambique?

5.3.1 Soft Systems Methodology process – Comparison of Conceptual models with the current situation.

5.3.2 Incorporating lessons learned from failures in the past and the HIS implementation process

5.3.3 Incorporating the experiences from similar implementations in other countries

5.1 The current state of the health information and knowledge management systems in the neglected tropical diseases sector in Mozambique

5.1.1 Soft Systems Methodology process – analysis of rich pictures

In analyzing the rich picture from the national planning meeting, it is clear that there are 3 distinct levels to the leprosy / NTD care system. The 3 levels were indicated by an eye symbol in green. The first is at community level where there is a social dynamic around the disease and its implications in the process of seeking help or coming to terms with possible physical or social complications that the disease may bring about.

The key actors here are the patient, wider family, traditional healer, and community volunteer. The latter is clearly the most important actor in this system, or where there are no volunteer it would probably be the healthcare personnel at the community clinic. As mentioned above, the community leprosy volunteers have a big role to play in the total service delivery, and there is a big network of them in Mozambique. Communication within this level is mostly by word of mouth but SMS messages and phone calls are also being used.

The second is at the clinical level with the interaction of the patient with the health services, and where the diagnosis needs to be made and treatment initiated.

Key actors here are the nurse at the community clinic, district supervisor, district clinical superintendent, management, and possibly also the laboratory technician and district pharmacy superintendent. The position of power here is with the district supervisor who has the clinical knowledge and access to the resources to diagnose and treat leprosy and its complications.

Actors communicate with each other within this level mainly by direct contact but also by phone or SMS messages.

The third level is the management level where there is a need for information and interventions need to be made to assure good service delivery on various levels.

Actors here would be the provincial supervisor, national level data analysts, national program managers, and other government institutions including the WHO. It is hard to say who is the dominant actor at this level as the interactions are much more complex and political in nature.

The communication channels here get a lot more complex but email and documents in various formats like Word and Excel are predominant. Phone calls and direct contact, like meetings are also important means for actors to coordinate.

Another important aspect coming out of the rich picture is the dynamic that exists where these three levels of care interact with each other, in order for that level to function and influence the outcomes of the bigger overall system and outcomes. These interaction levels were often a choke point or an area of conflict influencing the functioning of the whole system.

Aspects identified during the process of creating the rich picture are summarized in the table below.

	Level 1 - Community	Level 2 - Clinical	Level 3 - Management
Apparent goal	Get help / answers to deal with what is happening to me.	Make the correct diagnosis and start treatment.	Get timely and correct information to know what is happening.
Actors	patient, wider family, traditional healer and community volunteer	nurse at the community clinic, district supervisor, district clinical superintendent, district management, laboratory technician, district pharmacy superintendent	provincial supervisor, national level data analysts, national program managers, other government institutions including the WHO
Communication channels	word of mouth, SMS messages, phone calls	direct contact but also by phone or SMS messages	Email., phone calls, meetings
Choke points or conflicts	Men more stigma Long time before diagnosis made. Community volunteer bypassing local clinic.	Clinic nurses bypassed Lack of knowledge and engagement on leprosy. District supervisor far from village – limited transport means. Lack of support from district management.	Lack of timely knowledge from provinces. Not sure how much medicines to order. Long time delays in ordering and distributing medicines. Doubts on quality of the data.

Table 8: Characteristics of the levels of care in the NTD care system in Mozambique

The rich picture from the national data analysis team unpacks a bit more of the processes happening at national level as an illustration of the functioning of the previous health information system. It shows the processes around receiving, compiling, analyzing, and the destination and use of that information.

The apparent goal of this system was to produce timely and accurate reports for the various meetings and interdepartmental steering groups where the information was consumed. They felt great pressure from these politically important meetings and frustration towards the provinces and districts who did not supply them with complete information when it was needed. There was an admitted lack of feedback mechanisms to the provinces and districts. Even though disease specific indicators would likely have formed part of the information presented to the Ministry of Health coordination meetings, there was a lack of any reference to program specific goals or the management of these disease trends. The goal was just to produce the information and pass it on to the next level.

Actors here were the national data managers, various health ministry coordination and planning groups and the WHO. Communication was mainly via Excel or presentation documents or predefined forms for the various coordination bodies.

From the above it would seem that each level in the leprosy care system has a different goal that seems unconnected to the others. Actors seem isolated from each other with each responding to the pressures from the actors in their part of the system, but without the perspective of shared overall program goals. The health information system is driven by data managers on national level, not with the goal to improve program indicators, but to supply a report to actors that have very little knowledge of the realities on the ground, and where the information seems to have little impact on the decisions and actions needed to influence the outcomes for the NTD care system.

Lessons learned from this section for future HIS integration and a better link to Knowledge management :

- Program goals and key disease indicators should be more apparent.
- Program goals should be shared between levels in the care system.
- Program goals should drive the information system data gathering and use.
- Key actors should be identified where information can influence key decisions to impact program outcomes.
- Feedback mechanisms should be created to target these specific actors with relevant

information at the right times.

- Engagement needs to be stimulated between the different levels of the NTD care system using the information to evaluate key program goals and indicators. This could form part of the monitoring and evaluation system.
- Mobile communication seems to be a common communication form between most actors in the NTD care system. Perhaps this could be better utilized to share information and stimulate debate.

5.1.2 Soft Systems Methodology process – Analysis of stakeholder interviews

The feedback from district and provincial supervisors was analyzed separately to preserve some particular local perspectives that they may have.

On the **district level** the responses from supervisors again highlighted the relationships between the various actors in the system. It is clear that the dynamics here influence the outcomes of the program greatly. The importance of community partners in diagnosis and the follow-up of patients came out strongly, as did a bottleneck around resources needed for the supervisor to maintain this network. Maintaining the community network was facilitated by the increasingly available communication means and cell phone coverage.

It seems like the role of the district supervisors is a very dynamic one, with many varied tasks and expectations from clinical work to management, health education and planning. This seems to be a likely risk factor, as the quality off staff here has a great influence on service delivery in the NTD care system. Many responses also indicated a lack of time and resources to do their job, and their dependence on other partnerships to work effectively. Most district supervisors are responsible for both the NTD and the TB programs in their district with TB often getting preference as they feel a greater pressure to meet objectives set by the TB program. From informal conversations with provincial supervisors, it seems like there is also a high level of staff turnover among the district supervisors. This, again, highlights a possible weak link in the chain for effective NTD service delivery.

In analyzing the perceived objectives of the NTD care system from the perspective of the district supervisors, it was clear that attaining disease related objectives and to thereby "Come to an end of these illnesses" stood out for them as the goal of their work. This is positive and creates an opportunity for motivating them and guiding their role with appropriate feedback and indicator information.

From the responses from provincial supervisors, and as can be expected, they relied much more heavily on communication resources to fulfil their role which is more one of coordination between national and district levels. Many of the provincial supervisors were also responsible for the provincial TB program, and again it was stated that the TB program is more demanding and receives more attention. Even though supervision and giving technical support to the district level is one of the key roles of the provincial supervisor, it seems like there is a gap here with a lack of transport, and a felt frustration from the provincial supervisor in getting the data that he needs for their reports. They also see the goal of their system as improving disease indicators, but there was very little mention of their role in building the capacity of the district supervisors as a means of attaining this goal. **This seems to leave an impression that the role of the provincial supervisors is merely a channel for data to the national level and that their role as a middle level manager is not very effective and has little impact on the program implementation at the district level.**

In comparing the frameworks of the district and provincial supervisors we can see that there are great similarities particularly in the resources used by both groups. It was interesting that both groups saw **communication channels as a major contributor to fulfilling their role.**

There was also a lot of overlap in the type of activities of the two supervisor groups with clearly more clinical activities for the district supervisors and more coordination and data gathering activities for the provincial supervisors, which makes good sense and helps to confirm the validity of the feedback received in the initial rich picture.

Both groups also identified a lack of funding/resources as a hindrance to the implementation of their roles, and both indicated that data gathering/feedback was an important aspect influencing the outcomes of their work-system.

In looking at the objectives of their work-systems or the transformation that they want to achieve through it, both groups indicated that to obtain program goals and indicators was paramount. The district supervisors clearly had a much wider scope of relationships related to achieving these outcomes from both the patient and the partners participating in bringing about this transformation.

This is probably also an indication that **district supervisors are a key role player in the overall service delivery system** that we are studying.

Lessons learned from this section for future HIS integration and a better link to Knowledge management :

- District supervisors are the main producers of data / information in the NTD care system, but likely the last to consume it or benefit from it.
- Data gathering and feedback were aspects highlighted by both groups of supervisors as essential for achieving the goals of their system. The health information and feedback systems need to be designed to take the needs and realities of the supervisors into account. (rather than principally the needs at national level)
- District supervisors are key actors determining the outcomes of the NTD care system.
- The role of district supervisor is very multi faceted and requires a high level of clinical and institutional knowledge making them key focus players for knowledge management interventions.
- The monitoring and support structures for district supervisors are very weak and needs to be strengthened on district level. Feedback from the HIS could be an essential component to give direction to this monitoring and support, focusing on program goals.
- Mobile communication is well used by all supervisors creating opportunities for a health information system to use this channel of communication.
- The role of the provincial supervisor needs to to re-assessed to better translate bigger program goals for district intervention and then to grow a wider program ownership and accountability on district level. They need to add more value.

5.1.3 Document analysis results

The first set of documents analysed was from the reports given by the provinces during the rollout of the information system. These reports mostly represent a summary of the NTD care system at the time of the rollout and is a reflection on the problems experienced and issues raised by the districts before the introduction of the new information system.

The second set of documents analysed was a conjunction of pilot study reports and partners meetings which captured a lot of the learning during the process of implementation of the new information system. In general the reports from the various provinces that was received during the rollout of the health information system, seem to support the rich picture that was generated at the beginning of the process.

5.1.3.1 District reports

In using the performance measurement framework as adapted by (Faisst & Resatsch, 2004) to get an indication of the effectiveness of the information and knowledge management systems in action, the following aspects are highlighted by the feedback received from provinces:

Knowledge base indicators (Class I)

There is a lot of questions on the quality of data coming from the NTD system in general. There seems to be a lack of notification protocol and standardized procedures. The data gathering system in the NTD care system seems not to be in use everywhere and primary data sources like clinic cards are not well filled in or organized. Verification of data do not happen in many provinces which again draws into question the quality of the knowledge base.

Intermediation and transfer indicators (Class III)

A common theme coming from the provinces indicating the health of knowledge transfer within the system is the **lack of feedback** reported between all levels. This is not only the case between the various levels in the NTD care system, but also within partnerships on the district level for instance where information is not shared and thus the impact of the partnership diminished.

Knowledge transfer in the form of training seems also to be a big need, as there are lack of knowledge on basic indicators and program goals. Skills in getting access to information for instance in using Excel was also highlighted.

Knowledge transfer seems to be a key determinant for the outcomes of the NTD care system as the program outcomes depends on the cooperation of various key partnerships on the national, district and community levels. Also because of the longer term nature of the disease indicators it is needed to have a collective agreed consensus of the situation and the agreed actions to move the system forward. Without this each actor determines their own goals which might not be the most needed at that point and resources gets spent less effectively. **The health information system needs to be strong in its ability to share information across levels**. Specific processes also needs to be build into the knowledge management system to generate shared interaction around the information in order to **create perspective and shared ownership and direction**.

Effect indicators on business results (Class IV)

The above-mentioned failures of the information system has the consequence to impede one of the key objectives of the program, which is to break the transmission of Leprosy. It does so in a very comprehensive way by blocking the whole NTD care system from the partnerships and detection phase, the diagnosis stage and the treatment stage. A good example is the frequent lack of MDT (Multi drug therapy) that paralyses the whole care system. One aspect that stood out again was the importance of the Knowledge management system for the **correct distribution of resources** (for instance medications) for the care system to achieve its goals. The new health information system should be able to help managers plan the resource distribution better and monitor the levels MDT on various levels.

5.1.3.2 Reports and meeting notes from the roll out process

The next section summarizes the learning captured during the roll-out of the new information system. The same knowledge management performance measurement framework was used.

Knowledge base indicators (Class I)

As a critical factor for knowledge management in the NTD care sector the issue of **data standards and consistency** comes out strong in this section. As there are many partnerships and users around the HIS, each with different expectations and information needs, it is very important to have agreed upon standards and indicator sets. Data from key contributors like the National statistical department is structured very differently from a population point of view in comparison to the health delivery structure as indicated by the health department. Various partners or programs also have different information needs which could lead to a patchwork approach to the design of the database or the needs of a department may change, adding more requirements as has now happened with the need for GIS data for the NTD department. To manage this it seems like a very structured and formal approach is needed to make sure these decisions are made at the right level with the needed oversight and longer term perspective to assure an integrated approach is followed.

Also highlighted is the development of **critical partnerships** with for instance the National Statistical department that have access to the most up to date and accepted GIS data source without which the mapping results would be highly questionable.

Cost indicators (Class II)

The main concern that came out of the study data in this area was around **sustainability**, in particular relation to the equipment used for data gathering by the various users in the NTD care system.

In the case of the health department there was still very little experience in using mobile devices in the hands of so many users and issues of where to place the responsibility for the care and security of equipment and data was still untested.

The need for proper **standards for equipment and protocols for the use and replacement (mobile device management protocols)** are however highlighted as a key factor that would influence knowledge management. **Policies and procedures to ensure data security and privacy** of health information of patients would also be needed.

Partnerships or at least lesson sharing with other departments like the TB department seems a logical approach in order to develop shared approaches and avoid duplication.

Intermediation and transfer indicators (Class III)

In order to maintain a network of users, devices and applications, it became clear that certain **shared centralized libraries and registers** were needed. This was important as the users were sometimes changed, SIM cards or phone numbers changed or users could install a different application than the one originally installed. A shared repository for applications were created with F-droid as well as a user and password register on Google sheets.

5.1.4 Analysis of the technology survey

This survey was done to at least give a rough estimation of the level of technology use of the main service providers in the NTD care system and if this would be a hindrance to introducing an Android based information system. From the survey it seems like the majority of District Supervisors (73%)

already had a smartphone and that the majority of them were also active on social media like WhatsApp and Facebook. This was also confirmed during the implementation process where nearly all the district supervisors were found to be very able to use an Android based phone, install software, and navigate the system easily.

This probably contributed a lot to increase the acceptance of the HIS platform and speed up the integration and training process as **users were already used to the interface**.

For community level NTD service providers it was found that they also had a good level of connectivity with nearly 60% of community volunteers having at least a basic phone and practically all health post nurses having a basic phone or 61% having a smartphone.

The good connectivity and use of mobile technology is probably a factor that would contribute positively to knowledge management in the NTD care sector, as it would enhance both data gathering and information sharing.

In summary we have a older established medical care system that has not adapted much even though the external environment has changed a lot over the past 15 years. It still maintained the **organizational and personnel structures** established at the onset of multi drug therapy almost 30 years back. From the rich pictures drawn by the leprosy caregivers we see that there are 3 levels of care but that there are very different goals and expectations in each of the care levels in the system. This leads to an **operational divide** in the whole system and breaks down the overall effectiveness of the system to reach its goal. This is further worsened by the **communication inefficiencies and a lack of feedback** and **sharing of goals between care levels**.

Still there is a growing awareness of the need to improve communication accompanied by a strong commitment from the national management team. This is also supported by the growth in the availability and use of mobile technology by all levels in the care system, which opens up new possibilities for this communication to happen.

5.2 What should the aims of the health information system be in the neglected tropical diseases care context in Mozambique based on the specific objectives of this care system

In order to understand how to better integrate a health information system in this specific context and to understand what knowledge management is to achieve for the NTD care environment, it is important to borderline the system we are working with more clearly and then to define specifically what the output for that system should be.

In this regard we refer back to the Soft Systems Methodology (SSM) approach and we now try to draw together our knowledge of the context and background from the rich pictures and the interviews with actors from the previous sections. We will try to first define what is the system we are working with using the CATWOE analysis and Input – Output diagrams, and then then we will try and draw a Root definition from this to help capture the objective of the system.

5.2.1 Soft systems Methodology process : Input – Output diagrams

As illustrated by the Rich pictures, the system can be looked at from different perspectives for instance from the patient point of view, the District supervisor or direct service providers point of view and that of the higher level management. Each would want something different from their point of view and would define success also differently. This is illustrated by input-output diagrams as defined below:

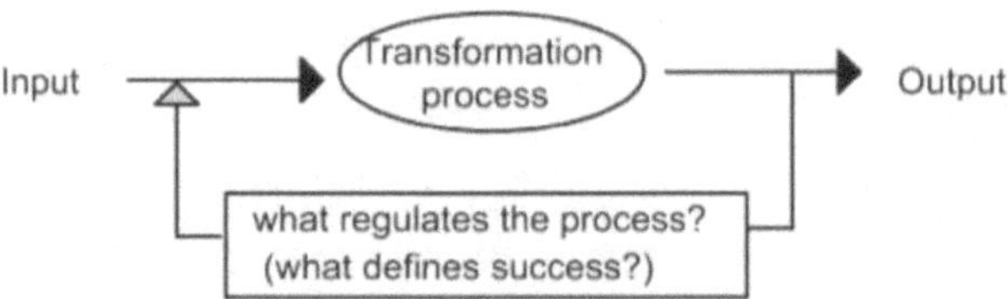

The following input-output diagrams was produced by actors from various levels in the NTD care system during planning and evaluation meetings in the course of the implementation process. Starting at the higher management levels in the system and drawing from the information from the actors in the NTD care system, the Input-Output diagrams initially looked like the following:

Data Analysts (National level)

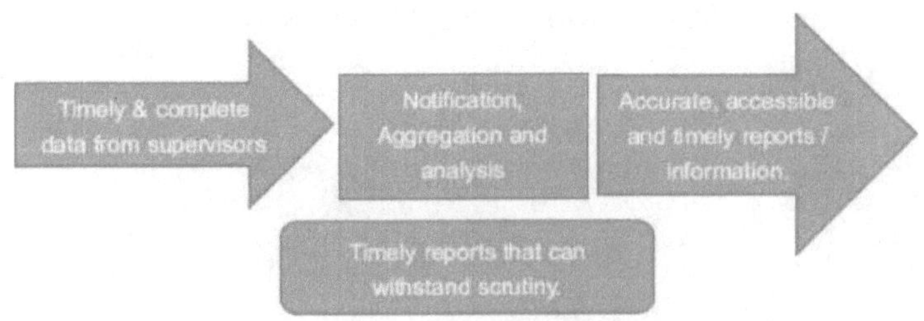

Illustration 18: Input-output model for national data analysts

Probably the biggest **transformation** that takes place for the Health information system is the **transfer of information** from one level to the next. This information can be defined as timely, accurate and complete leprosy case information that is received by the appropriate levels in the NTD care structure.

If it was just about installing a case notification system, this is probably where the exercise would end, but from the demands of the NTD care system as expressed by the different stakeholders below, that knowledge now needs to be put to work in specific ways to meet these demands.

Management level (national and provincial)

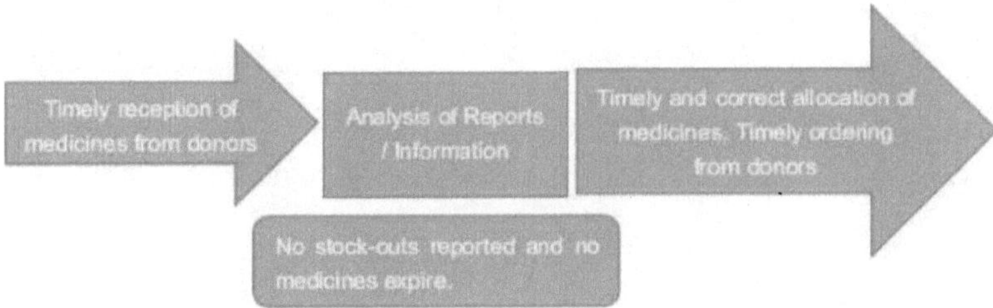

Illustration 19: Input-output model for national management

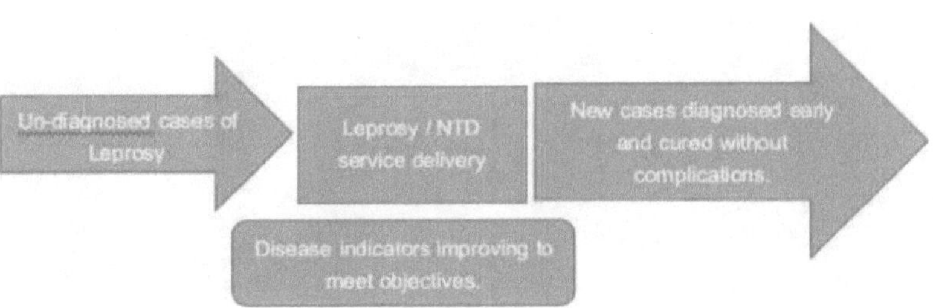

Illustration 20: Input-output model for national and provincial actors

Program implementation level (provincial and districts as well as patient)

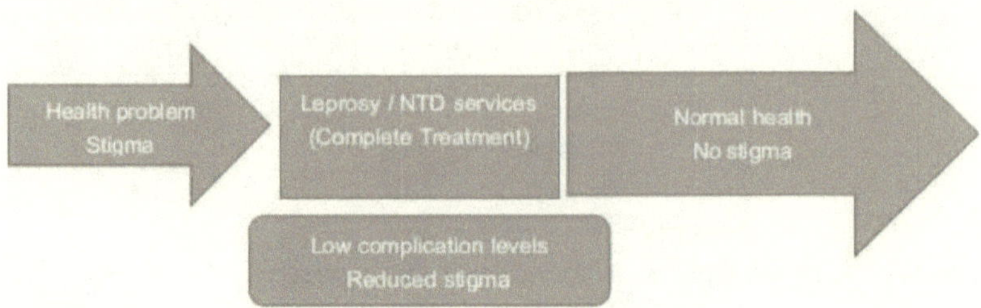

Illustration 21: Input-output model for district care providers

The above Input-Output diagrams represent some of the expressed expected transformations that different stakeholders have for the system. While the first, which is more in line with the needs of the data analysis team, is basically the transfer of information up the ladder, the other stakeholders in the system have a need for the information to be transferred back down again probably in an analysed and compacted form at certain times or on demand.

During a partner meeting after the pilot study, the partners was asked to do a CATWOE analysis and define what they saw as the goal of the system. They came up with the following CATWOE analysis and root definition:

Customer:	NTD managers and service providers
Actor(s):	District Supervisors
Transformation:	Notification, Aggregation and analysis of data. Registration and notification of data > Quality and timely information on indicators for various levels
Weltanschhaung *aka* **Worldview: (Why Bother...?)**	Good quality information is needed for resource allocation decisions and monitoring.
Owner:	Health Ministry / NTD Dept.
Environment:	Financial constraints Technical Requirements of the system, e.g. integration in the current health information system. Longer term maintenance and upkeep Cost-Benefit User participation and access Equipment upkeep, costs and access constraints Information should conform to WHO set indicators and program parameters

Table 9: Initial CATWOE analysis done by NTD service partners

The **root definition** as defined by the group was the following: A system owned by the health ministry with the objective to improve the health of people with NTDs/leprosy through data gathering, integrated in the National Health Information System by SDs and nurses, taking into consideration the environmental constraints to influence the decisions made, and actions taken at different levels that could influence the treatment outcome of the NTD program.

The **transformation** as defined by the group was very similar to that of the data analysis team on national level, namely the transformation of data to quality and timely information through the notification, aggregation, and analysis of data.

It seems however that the voice of program managers lower down in the NTD service delivery system is not sufficiently incorporated, as the transformation that they were envisaging was more related to the outcomes of the system for the patients, that is, the timely treatment of diagnosed cases

and the correct allocation of medicines. This further reinforces the observation that there is an **operational divide** between the national team and the NTD care givers at a district level.
The simple availability of information would probably already go a long way in addressing the Knowledge Management needs of the system, but there still seems to be a missing link between the information being available and appropriate actions being taken. Using the KM performance framework wording, the availability of information would address the knowledge base (Class I) and some aspects of the inter-mediation and transfer indicators (Class III) , but would still leave great gaps in addressing the contribution of knowledge to the final outcomes of the system (Class IV) and the cost effectiveness of interventions (Class II). Even though the Class I and Class III aspects are very important, it is the outcomes for the NTD care system and the efficiency that should probably be the drivers of the system as well as the definers of the knowledge elements (indicators) into which the system needs to feed.
In that regard, it seems necessary to define two systems with two key transformations in order to keep the system definitions more simple, and also to make sure enough emphasis is placed on the effectiveness and efficiency aspects of the NTD knowledge management system.
The following Input-Output diagrams give us an indication of the second transformation needed that addresses more the needs expressed by the District supervisors:

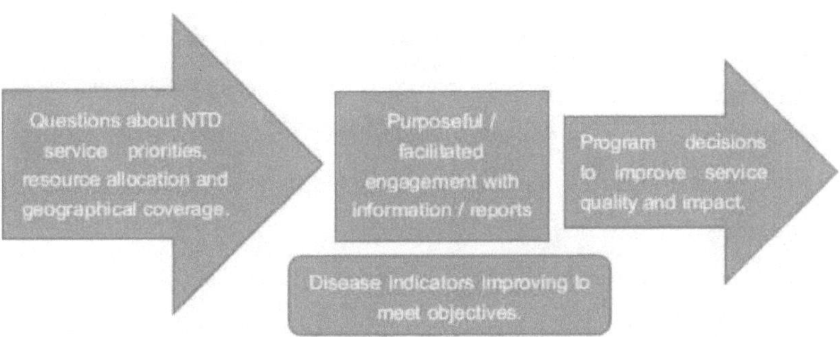

Illustration 22: Input-output model supporting program decision making

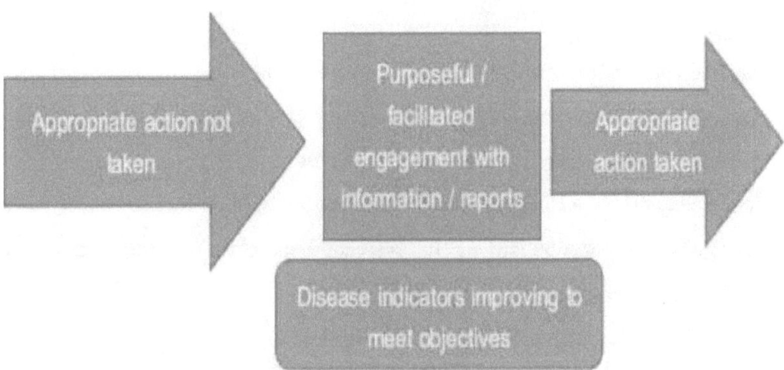

Illustration 23: Input-output model supporting program objectives

The **transformation** can probably be defined as some form of facilitated engagement or **knowledge appropriation** that takes ignorance to inquiry, questions to decisions, and required actions from not taken to taken at the appropriate time. Although this seems a difficult transformation to define and measure, it also seems like a necessary barrier to push in order to improve knowledge management within the NTD care system, and likely other similar systems also.

This is also supported by other feedback from the study of, for instance, the engagement levels described by the rich pictures. This type of transformation is strongly linked to the basic management functions of the NTD care system and the key engagement level there would likely be between the district and provincial program managers, which were also highlighted by the rich pictures as a weak spot. The provincial managers, that have a better overview of the situation and indicator trends, need to stimulate this engagement with the information among district supervisors and set goals for action.

The feedback from the document analysis also highlighted the need for the system to share knowledge across levels within the system and create shared ownership and direction, which will also support realization of this transformation.

In summary we have thus far identified two main transformations necessary to improve the knowledge management within the NTD care system, which are:

1. **transfer** of timely, accurate and complete leprosy case information between levels
2. knowledge **appropriation** by relevant stakeholders

Thus, the implementation of a Health information system in the NTD service context in Mozambique needs to take factors into account relevant to these two transformations in order to improve knowledge management in this context.

These two factors can also be seen in the context of the knowledge management performance framework we have been using. For instance, the **transfer** of accurate and timely knowledge is very much related to the knowledge base indicators (Class 1) as well as the intermediation and transfer indicators (Class 3). The knowledge **appropriation** factor is related to the cost indicators (Class 2) and the effects / impact indicators (Class 4) where the efficiency and effectiveness of the program is influenced by the way the knowledge is influencing programs outcomes and interactions between actors.

Taking these transformations as a starting point we can now follow the Soft Systems Methodology process and use the CATWOE analysis to define a root definition for these 2 systems.

5.2.2 Soft Systems Methodology process – CATWOE analysis and Root definitions

Transformation: transfer of case information

Customer: (C)	NTD managers
Actor(s): (A)	District Supervisors
Transformation: (T)	transfer of timely, accurate and complete leprosy case information between levels
Weltanschhaung *aka* **Worldview: (W)** **(Why Bother...?)**	Good quality information is needed to create reports and support management decisions and outcomes.
Owner: (O)	Health Ministry / NTD Dept.
Environment: (E)	Difficulties in verifying data quality. Communication barriers between levels. Technical Requirements of the system, e.g. integration in current health information system, longer-term maintenance and upkeep. Financial constraints > Cost-Benefit User participation and access. Equipment upkeep, costs and access constraints. Information should conform to WHO set indicators and program parameters.

Table 10: Revised CATWOE analysis for knowledge transfer in the NTD care system in Mozambique

5.2.2.1 Root Definitions for the information transfer system :

A System owned by O to do W by A by means of T given the constraints of E in order to achieve X for C:

A system owned by the NTD department to support management decisions through the transfer of quality case-based information by the District Supervisors in order to make timely and accurate information accessible to different levels of stakeholders. The system needs to be integrated into the existing National Health Information System and should be sustainable, taking into consideration the maintenance requirements, and end user adoption and usage costs.

__A system to do X, by Y in order to do Z__: **(X – What the System does , Y – How it does it , Z – Why it is being done)**

A system to produce meaningful and timely reports/information accessible to different levels of stakeholders through the transfer of quality case-based information by the District Supervisors in order to improve the outcome for people with NTDs in Mozambique (as defined by the program indicators)

Transformation: knowledge appropriation

Customer: People with Leprosy

Actor(s): Supervisors, healthpost nurses and community partners, NTD data analysts (NTD service providers)

Transformation: Purposeful / facilitated engagement with information / reports > appropriation of the knowledge.

Questions about NTD service priorities, resource allocation and geographical coverage > appropriation > Program decisions to improve service quality and impact.

Weltanschhaung *aka* **Worldview: (Why Bother...?)** Information needs to purposefully guide program and resource allocation decisions in order to improve health outcomes as reflected in the program indicators.

Owner: Health Ministry / NTD Dept.

Environment: Cost–Benefit

Resource constraints of the service providers to act on information.

High personnel turnover.

Table 11: Revised CATWOE analysis for knowledge appropriation in the NTD care system in Mozambique

5.2.2.2 Root Definitions for the knowledge appropriation system :

__A System owned by O to do W by A by means of T given the constraints of E in order to achieve X for C:__

A system (of reports, feedback loops and engagements etc.) initiated by the NTD Department to guide program decisions and resource allocation by the NTD service actors through purposeful appropriation of NTD health information in order to improve health outcomes for people affected by leprosy as measured by the program indicators.

<u>A system to do X, by Y in order to do Z:</u> (X – What the System does , Y – How it does it , Z – Why it is being done)

A system to improve appropriate program decisions/actions by NTD service providers by promoting the appropriation of NTD health information in order to improve health outcomes for diagnosed and un-diagnosed patients with leprosy.

The above system root definition formulations were based on standard system definitions used in the SSM process. Two different versions were used just to try and look at the system from slightly different angles to make sure the essence was captured.

In both the above sets of Root definitions we see that the owner and the main actors are basically the same groups. The main difference is the customer for which the system delivers the transformation. In the first system related to the transfer of case-based information, the flow is basically upwards towards the higher levels of the service hierarchy. The second system has a downwards orientation where the knowledge has to come down in an appropriate form to the level of each service provider in the service chain and then be used appropriately as guided by the program objectives.

5.2.3 Soft Systems Methodology process – Conceptual models

The next step in the SSM process would be the development of conceptual models based on the above two sets of Root definitions. The conceptual models helps us step into a systems-thinking context for a moment and try to define the most ideal way for this system to achieve the transformation that is intended as defined by the root definition.

Conceptual Model (Transfer of information):

1. Verify quality / completeness of primary data.
2. Notify / register / correct the data.
3. Verify aggregate data quality and completeness.
4. Disseminate timely reports / information.
5. Manage user adoption and proficiency.
6. Maintain the system infrastructure.

7. Monitor and manage system performance [1-6].
8. Continually develop and improve the system.

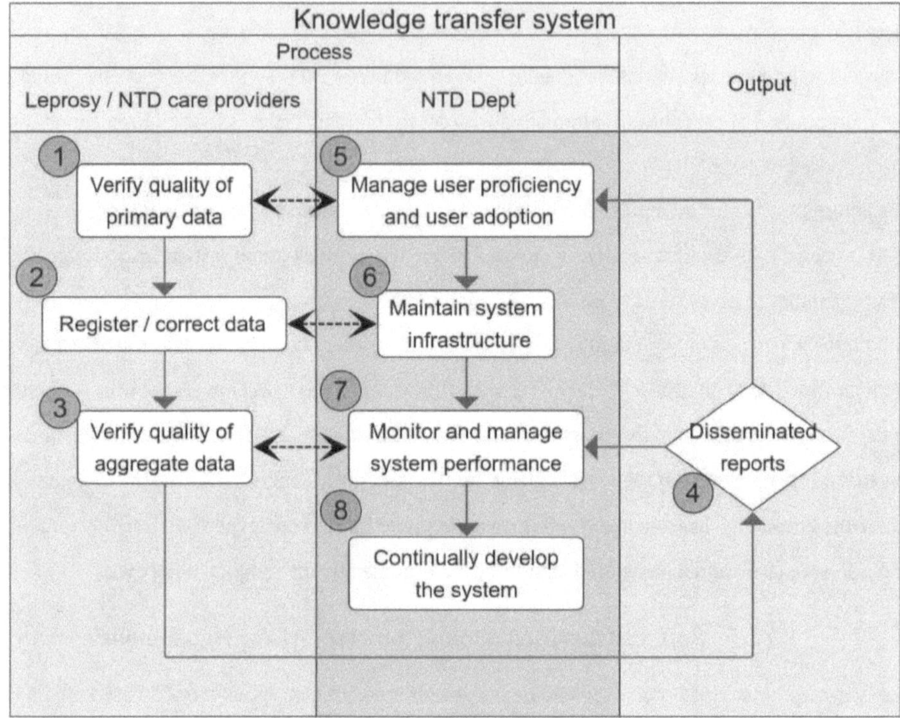

Illustration 24: Conceptual model of NTD knowledge transfer system

Conceptual Model (knowledge appropriation):

1. Define indicator goals and parameters for specific locations.
2. Identify and prioritize actors outside of parameters.
3. Engage with actors on the situation and desired outcomes.
4. Actor develop a plan of action to correct the situation.
5. Validate the action plan developed by the actor.
6. Monitor and manage system performance [1-5].

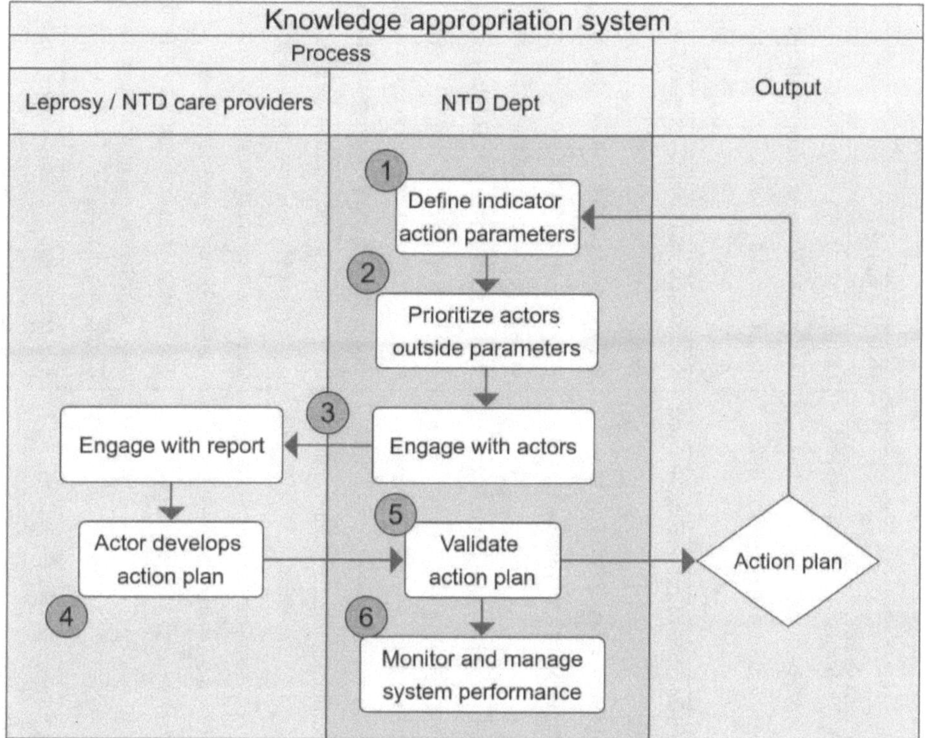

Illustration 25: Conceptual model of NTD knowledge appropriation system

5.3 What could a better model for knowledge management look like in the real world neglected tropical diseases context in Mozambique?

5.3.1 Soft Systems Methodology process – Comparison of conceptual models with the current situation.

In order to bring the conceptual models back into the light of the real world NTD care situation in Mozambique, we can use the following matrix to compare them to the actual situation by also using the data from the previous situation analysis sections.

Conceptual model activities	Does it exist?	How is it done?	How is it judged?
Verify quality / completeness of primary data. (Patient diagnosis and treatment card)	Partial	The person making the diagnosis fills in a standard patient treatment card. The quality depends a lot on the quality of training provided to the person filling in the treatment card.	During supervision visits the patient card is verified and where possible compared to the patient and patient treatment card.
Notify / register / correct the data	Yes	Information is filled into a Notification Register book kept in each district. With the introduction of the new DHIS2 based system the notification is made electronically on a tablet.	Supervision visits would compare the Register with clinic cards. In the case of the electronic registers, confirmation of notification is received immediately with an internet connection.
Verify aggregate data quality and completeness	Partial	In the previous paper-based system this could happen during a trimester verification meeting of supervisors. This does not happen in most provinces, however. Provincial supervisors did not have a practical way to verify the aggregate numbers sent to them by the district supervisors. In the new electronic system, the aggregation is automatically done by the database, both the district and provincial supervisors can view the same aggregate data.	Having access to the data does not imply that actors are using it. Usually the provincial supervisor would look at the aggregate data received from districts and would question the district supervisors if something seemed out of place. Indicators can be verified from the registers during supervision visits. The national statistical team would verify the completeness and timeliness of the information received.
Disseminate timely reports / information	Partial, not timely	Information is aggregated by supervisors from registers for trimester reports on indicators. These	The consumers of the reports were mostly at a national level, who judged the

		reports are compiled by the provincial supervisor and sent to the national office. In the new system the indicator reports are reflected in dashboards available to users or can manually be extracted from the database. Reports are not distributed to other district or provincial directors or medical supervisors routinely.	timeliness and quality of the information. The use of the reports was mostly not linked to clear program outcomes.
Manage user adoption and proficiency of the system.	Partial	Pressure from the national level to send data. Supervision visits. Training done sporadically. Some phone credit is occasionally sent to system users.	In the paper-based system the provincial supervisor usually had an idea of the relative competence of the district supervisor. In the electronic system the database can indicate which supervisors are not using the system or where there are many errors in the data sent.
Maintain the system infrastructure.	Partial to None	Register books are, in general, very old and seldom replaced. Provinces usually photocopied patient cards. Aggregate information shared by Excel sheets. The new DHIS2 based system is mostly maintained by the national Health Department but limited protocols and procedures exist for infrastructure maintenance and replacement (e.g. tablets)	There is no national systems audit in place, at least not for the NTD service sector, and there are few if any protocols in place to guide this.

Define measures of performance [1-6]	Partial	Standard indicators defined by WHO. Few National targets. Few national protocols or standards in place. Supervisions from National and Provincial levels. No system audits done.	Compared to International trends and standards. Best practice guidelines. National protocols (if in place). Best practice guidelines.
Continually develop and improve the system	Partial	Internal capacity growing but often still dependent on outside developers. No routine system reviews in place.	User reviews and system audits. Performance measurement results.

Table 12: Comparison of knowledge transfer model to current situation

From the above analysis of the knowledge transfer system, quite a few proposals can be gleaned that could positively contribute to improvements in knowledge management for the NTD care system by improving the knowledge transfer and quality. These are mostly aspects that are not in place or that are not functioning effectively:

- Ensure that service providers doing the diagnosis of leprosy are well trained and that primary data is well captured.
- Have standard procedures in place to verify the quality of primary data routinely.
- Ensure that the most effective and efficient system are used for the knowledge transfer (notification) step. Electronic tools seem to have clear advantages above paper.
- Define clear standards for data quality.
- Have a centralized electronic case-based register and do aggregation automatically.
- Build in verification procedures into the notification process. (Do not accept a notification if the data standards are not met)
- Ensure that program indicators and objectives are agreed upon and clearly defined.
- Define the information needs and timelines for each level of the NTD service chain with a clear link to the NTD program indicators and objectives.
- Create easier access to the relevant information for each level of NTD service provider. (edg. dashboards, tables and charts, indicator trends, etc.)
- Define a protocol for a national (and or district) information / systems audit of the NTD health information system and implement it.
- Define protocols for hardware and software specifications as well as maintenance and replacement procedures.
- Develop a training strategy and tools for system users, taking into account high staff turnover, resource constraints, and lower device exposure. Include training on the protocols and procedures defined for the system.
- Introduce indicators and procedures to measure the use of the system by especially the district supervisors and actively manage their participation including feedback mechanisms for system improvement.
- Actively feedback learning from systems audits and user responses to the continued improvement of the system as measured by the predefined objectives and changing program

needs.

For the knowledge appropriation system, the same matrix format was used to do a real-world comparison:

Conceptual model activities	Does it exist?	How is it done?	How is it judged?
Define indicator goals and parameters for specific locations.	No	When indicator levels cross certain predefined thresholds there should be red flags raised. This should be done automatically and visually by the HIS. National parameters not officially defined. No specific goals for provinces and districts defined.	Standard international indicators exist as well as expected objectives for these indicators. Local standards can be defined.
Identify and prioritize actors outside of parameters	Partial	No official parameters exist. Sometimes districts or provinces are perceived to have indicators outside of the norm, but this is mostly lightly defined and not followed up.	Locally defined indicator goals based on international standards.
Engage with actors on the situation and desired outcomes.	Partial	Only a few provinces have a trimester meeting where data is gathered and indicators discussed. Basic disease indicators included in district, provincial, and national health reports, but engagement is sporadic. Few engagement opportunities across levels in the service delivery chain.	The success of this activity could be judged by the level of engagement and ownership shown by the service providers and evidenced by action plans.
Actors develop a plan of action to correct the situation.	Partial	Provincial supervision plans exist probably in most provinces and districts. Supervisions are limited by lack of resources often. Where there are external funding partners (ILEP members) active in a Province, there are action	A national strategy with guidelines for provinces.

		plans and more awareness of indicators. In other provinces without this support this is lacking. The formulation of a national strategy started in 2015 but was never completed.	
Validate the action plan developed by the actor.	Partial	Results of activities shared during national coordination meetings where provinces are present. Provincial and district plans seldom shared or discussed.	Shared responsibility and accountability are based on national objectives. Reports from meetings and supervisions.
Monitor and manage system performance [1-5]	Partial	National Leprosy and NTD meetings on a yearly basis where provinces have to give report of what was done. Discussion on the level of activities rather than on indicators and strategies.	System audits or strategic reviews.

From this analysis of the knowledge appropriation system, the following proposals can be made to improve knowledge management within the NTD context:

- Create a national indicator framework and agreed upon indicator levels.
- Create feedback loops and ways to "flag" or highlight indicators that cross certain levels.
- Identify key actors, stakeholders and decision makers that would influence decisions in the NTD service delivery chain.
- Determine the appropriate content, timing and communication form for each key actor and seek ways to disseminate the information accordingly.
- Create forums of engagement either physically or virtually between actors of different levels in the system.
- Define an active monitoring framework where a response is required from key actors that received information.

5.3.2 Incorporating lessons learned from failures in the past and the HIS implementation process

In the previous section we concluded that for the system to attain its objective as described in the Root-definition produced by the owners of the system there are two main transformations that need to be achieved, namely knowledge transfer and knowledge appropriation. We have also formulated two conceptual models and compared them to the current reality in order to see what could be done to move closer to the ideal situation.

Referring to the history of previous information systems implemented in this context and applying the learning gained during the new health information system implementation process, we now need to further verify the above models. This will further give us an indication if this is a realistic approach and if we learned any further lessons as part of the action research approach. We further need to see if these lessons give us any more insight into which factors are more important to improving knowledge management in this context.

As stated previously, the knowledge management indicators in the framework adapted by Faisst and Resatsch (2004) seem to link well with the two factors of knowledge transfer and knowledge appropriation. The lessons learned was arranged accordingly in the following table:

Knowledge transfer	Knowledge appropriation
<u>Knowledge base indicators</u> Need for a single centralized database. Ways to verify the data quality should improve. Real time data input and analysis is needed. Data needs to be kept securely. Standardization of data sets needed. A verified and maintained GIS database is a key component for mapping. Certain partnerships are key to the success of the system and may need to be at an inter-departmental level to be sustainable, for instance	**<u>Cost indicators</u>** The total cost of maintaining a HIS should be taken into consideration (including meetings, etc.). The ability to capture data online and offline saves costs of connection and time. An equipment reference guide is needed indicating the minimum technical specifications of the equipment needed for the system. Terms of reference for the use and repair or replacement of equipment is needed.

Knowledge transfer	Knowledge appropriation
GIS data maintenance or similar programs like TB. A user and equipment register proved useful for coordination and maintenance.	Policies for Mobile Device Management needs to be drawn up and implemented. Users on their own initiative are able to find local solutions to issues for instance internet connectivity. To be more sustainable, clear terms of reference and description of responsibilities are needed for all actors in the system.
Intermediation/transfer indicators Access to data at all levels is a key ingredient to improve data quality and use. User friendly interface for users to input and access data. Feedback to district supervisors needed. Low internet speed and availability needs to be taken into account.	**Effects / Impact indicators** A flexible step-wise rollout process of the HIS involving the same team with frequent reviews of the outcomes proved very useful for learning and enabled improvements to be implemented sooner.

Table 13: Lessons learned from past failures and the implementation process

In the above analysis it seems that the factors at the base or foundation of the system, as well as factors that determine efficiency (cost indicators), dominate in the learning and feedback received from the implementation process. Examples of these factors include policies, protocols, procedures for the quality and upkeep of the database, and requirements of equipment. Also of note were key partnerships that added a lot of value. The message here is probably that these **foundational aspects are key to the management of knowledge within the system.** The same type of aspects are also mentioned in the MAPS toolkit (World Health Organization, 2015). In the MAPS toolkit, the emphasis is more on sustainability and scaling but the key is probably to try and build-in these important aspects from the start, or to at least build-in a process for them to be developed when enough learning and experience has been gained to give greater perspective of what is needed for the system. It was clear during the development and rollout process that the health department had little knowledge and experience in these foundational aspects of the knowledge management system as we could not demonstrate many examples from other departments or programs to use as a start for developing them for this program. It was important for the appropriation of this knowledge and learning to happen at some time during the process of implementing the HIS. The action learning process that followed during the implementation of the information system has contributed to many small and big improvements that were made, especially to the platform itself and the implementation process. There was not, however, sufficient time built in, especially towards the end of the roll-out process, to reflect on the more foundational issues and create or update policies and procedures accordingly. It seems a key learning that **processes need to be built into the HIS implementation process for knowledge and learning to be appropriated and translated into practice** according to the local context and circumstances. This seems to resonate well with what Jose Leopoldo Nhampossa (2005) also found when examining the integration process of health information systems in Mozambique. He also referred to gradual change strategies and mediating processes to enable participatory processes in the integration process. This appropriation should extend not only to the user platform and information system itself, but also to the more foundational and cost issues as they are highlighted during the process.

Although the above refers more to appropriation of knowledge during the initial implementation process of a new health information system, it is probably also relevant for the continued monitoring and evaluation of the information system and the processes that would support its continued development and maintenance in achieving its objectives. Also, these more foundational issues like policies would also need a revision from time to time.

When looking at the knowledge management maturity road map as defined by Robinson, et al., (2006), we can probably speculate that the system is at the second (uptake) of the 5 stages. Some goals are being established and some strategies are being explored. There are however a lot of basic issues like policies and protocols that still need to be addressed as well as issues related to sustainability, like equipment maintenance, where there is not a practical plan yet.

When taking into account the examples of unsuccessful attempts to implement some form of electronic health information system for leprosy in the smaller endemic countries like Mozambique, the question arises if it is realistic to expect these systems to be successful at all. Especially as these countries are weak in many of the basic elements needed for greater knowledge management maturity as highlighted above. The relatively low disease burden of Leprosy in these countries would further make it difficult to secure the needed political and financial investment to increase the possibility for these knowledge management systems to be maintained and sustained for the long run.

5.3.3 Incorporating the experiences from similar implementations in other countries

The process up till now has given us feedback of the actors in the NTD care system through the analysis of the rich pictures and additional information from the context data and interviews with various stakeholders in the system. From this we developed root definitions and conceptual models with some degree of verification by the users, thought this could probably have been more if time had allowed. The feedback received during the pilot and roll-out processes have helped to ground the learning further in the realities of the situation.

We now try to incorporate the lessons learned from other similar countries implementing similar systems as summarized in the Expert Interviews section above, to see if their experiences confirm the learning until now, and if they have further perspectives that could be incorporated. The same table structure, as above, was used.

Knowledge transfer	Knowledge appropriation
Knowledge base indicators Strategic thinking / planning for program goals that the HIS must support. Users should be involved in the design of the system. System functions within defined protocols and structure defined centrally. Documentation and detailed manuals available.	**Cost indicators** Important to create self-motivation among users for the system to run. Users often assume the cost of internet connection. Policies and procedures exist to control equipment and replacement. Equipment is insured > can be replaced if lost.
Intermediation/transfer indicators Tools that are easy to use promote data use. Wide participation in seeing the information Dashboards, which should be easily accessible. Data from the system needs to be used in reports and feedback back to the senders. Centralized training is followed by a Train the Trainer model and then monitoring and evaluation processes.	**Effects / Impact indicators** Training can promote the use of data by users. A scorecard system that can quickly flag something visually when action is needed. Integrated Disease Surveillance and Response guidelines > This helps to give staff thresholds for interpreting the data and taking action. Feedback loops at the lower facility level. Reports based on aggregated data from the system helps change behavior.

Table 14: Lessons learned from the Zimbabwe example

From the example of Zimbabwe, we see many more indicators on the impact side of knowledge management, for instance disease response guidelines, and a scorecard system to help actors translate the information to action. Also, on the aspects related to knowledge transfer, such as the functioning of dashboards and the use of data in reports, there are also indications of much more maturity in the system. It seems like the foundational aspects like policies and procedures are already in place and are being applied so less energy is spent on these aspects in the system.
When again looking at the maturity roadmap defined by Robinson, et al., (2006) we can find much

more evidence of maturity that would put the Zimbabwe example somewhere between the Expansion (stage 3) and the Progressive (stage 4) stages.

Some specific learning points that stand out include the **importance of self-motivation on the side of the actors to use the system**. This was seemingly developed by a combination of incentives for users but also having clear job descriptions and having a user-friendly interface. Users seem to have been involved during the design of the system and are being continually supported by a training and a monitoring system. It also seems like the information gathered by the users is being used and they perceive the feedback and impact of the data that they contribute. The **buy-in of the users** and having them taking ownership of the data and information seems to be a very positive contributor to the success of the system.

The other aspect that stands out was the use of a balanced scorecard system to help users flag issues in the program and take the appropriate action. It seems like some **Integrated Disease Surveillance and Response guidelines** were used in setting this up. This aspect, along with how the aggregate data reporting system is used, seems to promote the knowledge appropriation function of the knowledge management system.

For the Ghana experience the same table format was used to structure the learning:

Knowledge transfer	Knowledge appropriation
Knowledge base indicators Health department have the capacity to evaluate their own needs and seek own solutions. Predefined operating procedures exist for the system. An elaborate framework of aligned policies and guidelines supports the DHIS2 setup. Policies and guidelines in place for equipment use and replacement. Yearly audits of the IT system on various levels.	**Cost indicators** Responsibility for Cost for routine access to the DHIS2 server (internet costs) are decentralized and facilities and districts. Training is more decentralized - on the job type training rather than centralized form of training. Planning and budgeting should happen at facility level and be based on data from the system and then put together at higher levels. The service data is linked to the Ghana Health Services objectives, to look at the burden of

Knowledge transfer	Knowledge appropriation
	diseases, plan accordingly, where resources are allocated.
Intermediation/transfer indicators Reviews stimulate the facility level staff to take ownership of their data and the consequences. Feedback sent down the line. Having access to data, visualizing it effectively and getting feedback stimulates ownership and use. The core person is to champion and promote the use of the system is on middle level management.	**Effects / Impact indicators** System of performance reviews on all levels based on DHIS2 data from system. Performance and appraisals need to be used to stimulate people to use the data.

Table 15: Lessons learned from the Ghana example

When again looking at the maturity road-map defined by Robinson, et al., (2006) it seems like the program in Ghana is not quite as far along as the example from Zimbabwe, but still probably at least a solid Expansion phase (stage 3).

The Ghana experience did not bring much new information to light, except maybe the comment on the **importance of the middle level management to promote the use of the system** and serve as champion. It also seems that their **system is well integrated**, that is, their planning, budgeting, and program objectives are well integrated and supported by their health information system.

6 Discussion and Conclusions

From the analysis above we can distill the following proposals for the implementation of a health information system able to support the knowledge transfer and knowledge appropriation aspects of the NTD knowledge management system:

6.1 Proposals to support knowledge transfer

1. The design and implementation of a health information system should happen within the predefined (and documented) **framework of adequate policies and protocols** so that standards can be assured, and compatibility improved. These include policies for data security and privacy, standards for indicators and data sets, mobile device management, and user management and training. As seen from the examples of both Zimbabwe and Ghana, having this framework in place and in use added a lot of value to the monitoring and evaluation system, and the longer-term sustainability of the information system.
2. A **single centralized database** makes data gathering and knowledge sharing much easier.
3. Ways to **verify the data quality from start to finish** should improve. This would start with good definitions of data elements and indicators and the standardization of data sets. It would also mean reviewing the appropriateness and quality of the primary data sources which could be paper forms or clinic cards. It would also include data verification steps or procedures during each transaction where data is passed from one level to the next, for instance automatic verification algorithms during electronic data capture, etc.
4. **Real time data input and analysis** is needed. The sooner the users can get feedback from the data they provide, the sooner data errors can be spotted and corrected, and the sooner the information can be appropriated. It probably also adds to a greater sense of ownership of the information provided.
5. **Data needs to be kept securely.** Data protection probably needs to be built into the planning early in the process but should be appropriate to the needs and local capacities to maintain it.
6. If the system needs to be able to do mapping, **a verified and maintained GIS database** is a key component. It is likely that some extra effort is needed, and partnerships created to get good data, and also to maintain it.
7. **Strategic partnerships can add a lot of value but need development and maintenance**. This could, for instance, be around the GIS data, or it could be with similar programs where synergy is possible, for example, TB and other NTDs. It is also necessary to see that for certain partnerships to be sustainable they need to be on a scale big enough to justify the effort and to add value to other actors that may be at the periphery.

8. A **user and equipment register** proved useful for coordination and maintenance. This is fairly simple to do but saves a lot of time when maintained centrally.
9. **Good access to data at all levels** is a key to improve data quality and use. This is not so easy to achieve, especially if more levels of users' needs are to be incorporated. Though, platforms like the DHIS2 system make it a lot simpler. It should however be planned for from the start of the project and should give preference to the lower level of actors who provide most of the data. Having good access to information is facilitated by having a user-friendly interface in the database application. It could also mean different things to different levels of users, for instance, appropriate technology, where the district supervisors would need a different type and have different connectivity options to that which the central NTD department may have. Data should also be packaged so that users can interact with it according to their specific needs, for instance the ability to sort or filter the data according to location or date. The DHIS2 dashboard system seemed to add good value.
10. **Feedback to district supervisors needed**. As we have seen, the district supervisors are the main sources of information and they have the most clinical contact with the patients and exerted the greatest influence on program outcomes. Feedback promotes ownership and use of the information, and should, where possible, link to program goals and indicators. As seen in the examples from Zimbabwe and Ghana, the feedback should come from the middle management level, above the district supervisors, and refer to their data, strongly pressuring them to take ownership of it.
11. Internet connectivity would be essential for the transfer of data, especially when implementing an electronic online database like DHIS2. It seems however like a more practical option to **delegate the responsibility for connectivity to the district level** and to allow district supervisors to find local solutions.
12. An **appropriate training strategy is needed** to support the continued implementation and running of the information system. It seems like a decentralized Train the Trainer model was mostly used by other similar programs.
13. The core person to **champion and promote the use of the system is at the middle management level**. In the case of the NTD care sector in Mozambique, this would be the

provincial supervisor. As stated earlier, the role of these supervisors needs to redefined. They need to be more than a channel of information from the district supervisors to the central level but should rather facilitate the use of the information by the district health departments, who in turn will link back to the district supervisors.

6.2 Proposals to support knowledge appropriation

1. In the light of the changing epidemiological situation on the Neglected Tropical diseases care sector, it is necessary that the national program **define the goals** for the system clearly and that the **strategical approach to achieving these goals is revised**. This will give direction, and focus the design and implementation of the knowledge management system.
2. It may also be necessary, as highlighted by the rich pictures, to revise the organizational structure of the care system and to **redefine the job descriptions** of the actors in the system. This will help these actors understand their role and support the appropriation of knowledge by them, in fulfilling their roles.
3. The **total cost of maintaining a HIS should be taken into consideration**. There seem to be many hidden costs that are not considered during the initial setup of a new information system, but if it is not budgeted for, eventually will erode the longer term sustainability of the system. These costs include meetings with stakeholders to sort out working procedures and protocols, regular systems audits, continued user training, adequate mobile device management, adequate data security and backups, the cost of internet connectivity, equipment maintenance and replacement etc.
4. The **ability to capture data online and offline** saves costs of connection and time. Especially in a context where internet connectivity is not always possible, it gives a lot flexibility to the district supervisors.
5. As also stated above, the system should function within the bounds of a **framework of policies, protocols and procedures** and these should be well communicated to the actors in the system. This should include clear terms of reference and a description of responsibilities, for all actors in the system. When these are clearly understood, it frees up the actors to take the necessary steps to ensure the continued functioning of the system. Other essential parts

that also need to be defined include an equipment reference guide detailing the terms of reference for the use and repair or replacement of equipment, and standards for mobile device management.

6. As seen from the example of Zimbabwe, when there is a high degree of **local ownership and a sense of shared responsibility**, users on their own initiative are able to find local solutions to issues, for instance internet connectivity. This sense of local ownership should be encouraged especially by having **people take responsibility for the data submitted by them** or their areas, and **making it visible**, for instance in reports and quality audits. The sense of ownership is also enhanced when they have good access to their data and local management are able to view the information. Ownership is also stimulated by decentralizing responsibility for cost of routine access to the DHIS2 server.
7. Adequate **training can promote the use of data by users**. This would likely include a breakdown of the basic indicators of the program as well as how to get feedback on these indicators for their level.
8. The examples from Zimbabwe and Ghana also highlighted the importance of a feedback system based on the program indicators and outcomes. When the system is able to **visually flag an issue that needs attention or action** based on some agreed disease surveillance and response guidelines, it could help to address issues sooner. These feedback loops should also include the lower levels in the NTD service chain.
9. The program monitoring and evaluation system should implement **performance reviews based on data from the system**. In the same way, service data and outcomes for program indicators should inform planning and the allocation of resources. Even though this may seem obvious, it is probably necessary to be very intentional about it.
10. Having a **flexible step wise roll out process** of the HIS, **involving the same team** with **frequent review of the outcomes**, proved very useful for learning and enabled improvements to be implemented sooner. It is also important to build-in time in the roll out process for this learning and adaptation process to happen.

The above summary of learning points for knowledge transfer and knowledge appropriation is a mixture of bigger picture issues as well as system elements and procedural factors. The learning can also be summarized using these groupings:

6.3 Bigger picture issues that support knowledge management

It is necessary to **adequately define the goals and strategy** of the care system at the start of the process. This will give greater direction to the whole design process of the information system. Leading from this would be a review of the **organizational structure and roles of the actors** in the system. At this stage it may be beneficial to look at the role of knowledge appropriation, before the elements of knowledge transfer is defined. What are the processes of learning and decision making that will move the system to achieve its goals, and which key relationships in the NTD care system will support this? What information would these actors need to support this engagement process and how can it be provided for them at the right time?

The design and implementation of an information system needs to happen within the bigger **framework of policies, protocols, and procedures** that is likely defined at national level. This is to ensure that standards are defined, and compatibility and sustainability improved, etc. Without this framework, the system is at serious risk of becoming outdated or unsustainable after a few years. It is thus necessary to look at the **total cost of implementing the system**, including the elements of policy frameworks, monitoring and system audits, equipment maintenance and continued training. It is important to assure that there is **sufficient capacity within the system for the continued maintenance and development** of the system after the initial design and implementation team are no longer on the scene.

Some **key partnerships may be needed** that fall outside the scope of the specific NTD program. These partnerships are however quite essential for the continued development and future of the information system, for instance the validation and upkeep of the GIS data used in the system, or other related programs like tuberculosis, or the team responsible for database maintenance. These partnerships need development and upkeep.

Connectivity to the internet is clearly important for a modern information system to function. There are, however, other ways to maintain this other than the total responsibility resting with the NTD program. This aspect can for instance be delegated to the district level or a high sense of ownership can be encouraged so that users take on the responsibility if the official mechanisms fail.

For the NTD care system in Mozambique, the key user is the district supervisor, and the **key champion is the provincial supervisor.** Provincial supervisors should be made aware of their role as champions and enablers in the knowledge management system. The early adopters would be key activists to also mobilize and train during the implementation process in order to get others to adopt the system over the long run (Braa et al., 2001).

6.4 Elements of the health information system that promotes better knowledge management

A **single centralized database** makes data gathering and knowledge sharing much easier.
Tools and procedures to **verify the data quality** from start to finish should be designed in.
Real time data input and analysis improves user acceptance and ownership of the data and results.
Adequate **data safety and security** policies and procedures would be necessary, especially in an environment with high stigma.
Where the internet connectivity cannot be guaranteed, the chosen platform should be able to capture data **online or offline**.
A verified **GIS database** and adequate skills in managing GIS data and integration would be a prerequisite if any form of mapping is to be used. It is also necessary to reflect on how the mapping data would be used afterwards to help define the level of detail and the way the locations are structured.
A **user and equipment register** is a small thing but very useful when needed.
A **mobile devise management** strategy and policy comes into play not only when the inevitable loss or breakdown of equipment happens, but links strongly also to the data safety policy.
A **friendly user interface** that **facilitates access to the data** elements and aggregate data for different levels of users. For instance, the system should allow for the verification of data by the actors that supplied the data.
Routine feedback mechanisms to provide reports or key information to key actors should be designed into the system. These should be routine and automatic where possible. Reports should be highly structured and **visual** to encourage engagement with the information. When there are indicators outside of the normal parameters, the system should automatically highlight them.

An initial and a **continued training strategy** is needed to maintain user capacity.

A **monitoring system** is essential to monitor not only the transfer of knowledge, but also the appropriation side of the equation. This could take the form of routine performance reviews based on data generated by the system.

6.5 Implementation process elements that contributed positively to the implementation

The **Soft System Methodology process** that was followed was useful in that it gave the opportunity to hear and incorporate the perspectives of all of the key system actors. The **action learning** approach also gave plenty of opportunity to incorporate lessons learned during the design and implementation process of the information system.

The **involvement of all related actors** in the design process of the health information system adds value in the longer term and probably contributes to quicker acceptance of the system. As theorised by the Actor Network Theory, the introduction of a new information system in the current NTD care network will affect the functioning of the whole network (Cresswell et al., 2010). The system will be strengthened and maintained to the degree that there are constructive engagement between actors (which includes the new technology) and new alliances are formed with the translation the new technology into a network of meaning and use (Alexander & Silvis, 2014). Practically put, for the new health information system to be accepted and adopted, it is important that the health department **help the actors understand its relevance to them and the costs and benefits involved**. It should also **stimulate engagement with the system** as much as possible to facilitate the creation of alliances of practice.

A **flexible step wise roll out process** of the HIS **involving the same team** with **frequent review of the outcomes** proved very useful for learning and enabled improvements to be implemented sooner. It is also important to build in time during the roll out process for the learning and adaptation processes to happen.

This study coincided with the design and implementation of a new health information system for the case managed neglected tropical diseases care sector in Mozambique. The aim was to incorporate lessons learned from the past, and to give the NTD care sector some more tools not only to gather data, but to translate the knowledge gained into better health outcomes for patients. For this reason, the following research question was formulated:

What factors would contribute to the successful implementation of a health information system for CM-NTDs in order to improve Knowledge Management within the wider NTD care system?

The study found that there were mainly two key factors that would contribute to better knowledge management within the NTD care sector in Mozambique and that needed to be kept in mind when designing and implementing a health information system in this context. These factors are adequate knowledge transfer and knowledge appropriation.

Knowledge appropriation, especially, could be wrongly perceived as an incidental outcome of a good knowledge transfer system, but it is crucial to reflect on appropriation at the start of the design process as it addresses many of the factors leading to health information systems failing. It can also help give greater context to the design of the knowledge transfer elements in the system, as it brings in the perspective of the users of the information system and their role in influencing outcomes for patients.

The study identified various overarching factors (big picture issues) as well as health information system elements and implementation process elements that contribute to improved knowledge transfer and appropriation in this context. For knowledge appropriation, some of the more important elements include the need for an appropriate policies and standards framework, as well as the need for processes to stimulate engagement with program results between key actors. Among others, knowledge transfer, included the need for data verification from start to finish, and appropriate access to data for all users in the system to accomplish this.

The study also proposed two conceptual models for knowledge transfer and appropriation in this context. These can serve as a basis for evaluating the real-world context in similar NTD care situations where a health information system needs to be implemented.

Lessons learned from the implementation process as well as the Soft Systems Methodology process could also contribute to similar implementation processes elsewhere.

6.6 Future research suggestions

During this study, the importance of knowledge appropriation was highlighted. Even though this may be the case, it still leaves us with many questions as to how this could be done in practice. This interface between knowledge, information systems and the human actors in the system brings the social and cultural aspects much more into play. Knowledge transfer seems much easier to design into a system and are much easier to monitor and control than would be knowledge appropriation. Even though appropriation may be difficult to delineate, the impact on the final outcome for patients is increasingly more apparent. For this reason it would be useful to understand knowledge appropriation from a theoretical and a practical perspective better.

The socio-technical interaction around appropriation brings to mind the actor network theory once again, especially around the aspect of agency. Agency roughly defined would be the ability to make a difference or influence other actors in the system. For knowledge appropriation this is of course very relevant, as we would want the key actors in for instance the NTD care system to have more appropriate agency and for them to apply that agency to improve outcomes for patients. If an actor has knowledge but limited agency, the usefulness of the knowledge is also defeated.
From the ANT point of view all actors in the system can have agency, including the non human components like information systems. The nature of this agency and the differences between machine agency and human agency is very much in flux (Jones, Rose, & Truex, 2005) especially as new technologies keep pushing the boundaries of this engagement. It might be an interesting topic of further research to explore how the agency of the human actors can be enhanced, but also how increasingly interactive and "intelligent" information systems can play a bigger role to enhance both knowledge transfer and appropriation and in so doing influence the outcomes for patients.

After the roll-out of the new NTD health information system came to an end and the dust started to settle, it quickly became apparent that the system can not be static if it is to be sustainable and relevant only a year later. This dynamic nature of innovation and how actors engage with and influence the elements and characteristics of it over time is a key component to its sustainability. As a followup study, it would be very useful to understand how this process of adapting, improving and restructuring has contributed to the success or failure of the system. It also seems important to learn how to integrate these adaptive processes and flexibility into a new technology that is being introduced to a system, especially as the institutional actors may not be quick adapters.

The NTD care sector and especially the leprosy care sector is one of the least developed and under financed. As seen from this study, there are many technical and institutional capacities necessary for a system to be implemented successfully and be sustainable. These capacities may be hard to come by in the typical environment where NTDs are found. A question that still remains and may warrant further study is whether a global approach to creating a basic shared electronic health information framework for leprosy and promoting knowledge management from this level is not more feasible and sustainable. Especially if bigger partners like the WHO were to maintain the basic infrastructure and provide it as a service to countries wanting to subscribe. The dynamic elements of translating such a framework to the local context, as repeatedly seen during this study, will have to be understood and planned for.

www.ingramcontent.com/pod-product-compliance
Lightning Source LLC
LaVergne TN
LVHW041100150826
845673LV00007B/1863
9783384228161